THE CINNAMON BOOK

By Emily Thacker

1

Published by:

James Direct Inc

500 S. Prospect Ave.

Hartville, Ohio 44632

U.S.A.

This book is intended as a record of folklore and historical solutions and is composed of tips, suggestions, and remembrances. It is sold with the understanding that the publisher is not engaged in rendering medical advice and does not intend this as a substitute for medical care by qualified professionals. No claims are intended as to the safety, or endorsing the effectiveness, of any of the remedies which have been included and the publisher cannot guarantee the accuracy or usefulness of individual remedies in this collection.

If you have a medical problem you should consult a physician.

Not For Resale

ISBN: 978-1-62397-022-2

Printing 12 11 10 9 8 7 6 5 4 3 2 1

First Edition   Copyright 2012   James Direct Inc

Table of Contents

A Letter from Emily

Dear Readers,

It is with great excitement that I come to you once again with another addition to our collection of natural home health remedy books. It is hard to believe the very first book in this series was brought to you nearly 20 years ago with the best-selling, *Vinegar Book*.

The Vinegar Book was the book that started it all, listing hundreds and hundreds of ways a simple bottle of vinegar could be used to transform the way we clean, eat, and particularly the way we treat both chronic and common health conditions and illnesses. Simple home remedies forever changed the way we viewed illnesses and the treatment of those maladies.

From there, we introduced new home remedy solutions such as garlic and baking soda, honey and tea, and even a new book on the amazing ways hydrogen peroxide can be used for better health. The basis of each book in this series was to introduce natural home health remedies into our everyday lives, and look at the research behind those remedies.

These books have always been a special treasure of mine, as I whole heartedly believe in getting back to the natural properties of health care as much as possible. It is with this thought in mind that I am proud to introduce to you the latest in my series of natural health books, *The Cinnamon Book.*

This book is particularly exciting to me, as the subject is a personal favorite of mine – cinnamon! Who doesn't love the wonderful aroma of warm cinnamon rolls baking in the oven on a crisp fall morning? Or what about the sweet fragrance of fresh cinnamon sticks steeping in a piping hot cup of tea? And who can forget the fun taste of cinnamon candies we enjoyed as children?

The mention of cinnamon goes back thousands of years, and even has several mentions in the Bible. Our great grandmothers used cinnamon as a way of stopping the pain of a aching tooth, and looked to cinnamon to soothe an upset stomach. Cinnamon and honey steeped in a warm tea was often given to fight a nasty cold. And many have sworn to the effectiveness of adding cinnamon to warm applesauce as a way of stabilizing blood sugar levels. Hundreds of uses could be rattled off counting the ways our grandmothers depended on cinnamon in years past.

But cinnamon is so much more.

Did you know cinnamon contains natural healing properties that can be used to fight against rising cholesterol rates, heart disease and even diabetes? Studies have shown cinnamon to be useful in dealing with boosting memory function and even easing symptoms of the common cold. It is high in antiseptic and antibacterial qualities making it ideal for treating infections and fighting bacteria. It is also a known anti-clotting agent and is oftentimes used as an anti-inflammatory remedy.

And the latest research is even more promising. New research studies are showing that cinnamon's amazing health attributes of being an anti-tumor agent as well as a known antioxidant that, when used properly, may be extremely effective as a possible cancer prevention agent. Scientists are excited about the many promising research results their research studies are beginning to bring to the field of medicine.

Unlike over the counter medications or drug store prescriptions, cinnamon is inexpensive to purchase in comparison to most drugs and is readily available. It is easy to store, lasts a long time, and simple to use. Cinnamon comes in various forms and its medicinal integrity stands up to being cooked to high temperatures. Did I mention cinnamon is delicious, too? Chances are, you probably have at least one form of cinnamon in your kitchen pantry right now.

Scientific trials also show cinnamon to be extremely effective in raising the body's natural metabolism to aid in weight loss. Not only does it speed up metabolism naturally, but it also works to stabilize blood sugar and insulin levels and lower harmful LDL ("bad") cholesterol numbers. All of this better helps the body shed inches and unwanted pounds.

In doing the research for this book, my primary consideration, as always, when bringing you natural health tips and remedies is:

- Can this do you harm?

- Is it safe to use?

- Is it time tested?

- What does the research show?

- What are the benefits?

- What (if any) are the potential downfalls?

- What information is most helpful to the reader?

In this book we will explore a multitude of ways this simple, fragrant spice can be used for better health and natural living. Far too many times we are too quick to reach for the latest drug or medication, without first exploring the simplicity of getting back to the basics. Pharmaceuticals, while often times necessary, can more times than not come with unwanted side effects and conditions that can be as bothersome as the reason we chose to take the medication in the first place. And, we are all much too familiar with the skyrocketing prices of medications these days.

Is this to say we should stop taking our physician prescribed medications altogether? Absolutely not. But, my hope for this publication is to act as a springboard between you and your family healthcare practitioner to give you alternatives to help you take control of your personal healthcare needs. Many of these remedies and plans should be discussed with your doctor to see if a more natural route of health care is a possibility for you. And, in this book you will find many suggestions and ideas for laying a solid, healthy living foundation in your life before trouble hits. Preventative action is always the best medicine. In *The Cinnamon Book,* you will find a treasure trove of actionable ideas that you can begin to use right now.

Not only will you read about simple home remedies ready for you to put use immediately, but we will also investigate some of the latest scientific research that is on the horizon. Some of these studies are showing very encouraging results for suffers of heart disease, Alzheimer's disease, diabetes and obesity, just to name a few.

And no book about cinnamon could possibly be complete without fantastic recipes to help incorporate cinnamon into your meal plans. We have tested countless recipes highlighting cinnamon's delightful flavor and aroma and now bring you the best in everything cinnamon — entrees, side dishes and flavorful desserts. In fact, we have dedicated an entire chapter to that incredible breakfast pastry we all know and love, cinnamon.

There is also a special section in the chapter entitled, Cinnamon for Weight Loss, that gives you a few low fat recipes to try and enjoy. It also helps explain the science behind using cinnamon as a metabolic enhancer and explores the much regarded Cinnamon Diet.

Many of the ideas explored in *The Cinnamon Book* are backed up with scientific data and research. Other suggestions are deeply rooted in folklore or handed down from generation to generation, from one family to the next. And, what works for one person's condition or ailment may not be right for another. You will find many of these suggestions very helpful, while other ideas may not be the best solution available for your particular problem. It is up to you, the reader, to decide which ideas will work best for you, in your particular circumstance or condition. It also presents a wonderful opportunity to work together with your health care provider in finding the best solution that is right for your life. And with exploring more natural ways to treat healthcare problems, we are placing healthcare back where it belongs – in your own hands.

As with any home remedy or before making regular use of any natural health or alternative treatment, be sure talk openly with your doctor. Keep in mind this book is an attempt to share information. And as with any treatment, cinnamon has its limitations. Be sure to use it wisely and always in moderation. Pay close attention to any warnings listed throughout the book, and heed all cautions presented by your healthcare physician.

So grab yourself a cup of warm tea — maybe even add a cinnamon stick or two - and join me in discovering the many amazing and wonderful uses for that simple, delicious spice we know as cinnamon.

And, as always, I welcome the opportunity to connect with you! Please feel free to write to me and share your own experiences with how you use cinnamon for better health. Have a wonderful cinnamon recipe to share? I would love to read it! Who knows, it may even end up in a future edition of one of my books!

I look forward to hearing from you and reading about all the personal uses you have found for cinnamon.

Wishing you all my best,

Emily

Wait! Before you read this book...

Want to get your Special Bonus? Because you've ordered this book from one of our online distributors (and not directly from us jamesdirect.com), they are not able to send you the FREE Bonus.

But, if you email James Direct with your confirmation receipt (after purchase) we will make sure you receive your Special Bonus booklet.

To receive your Special Bonus please do this: email us at customerservice@jamesdirect.com and write in the subject line Bonus Dept CIN124.

Then in the body of the email please provide us with your first & last name and postal address of where we should ship your bonus booklet. Also, please specify if you want it emailed to you or if you'd like an actual booklet shipped to you.

CHAPTER ONE
Introduction

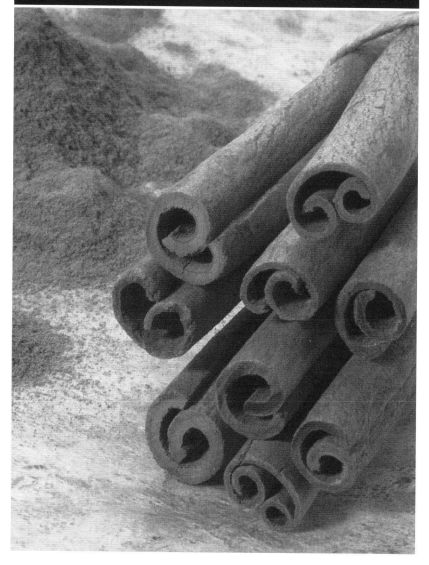

Thank you for your interest in *The Cinnamon Book*, the latest in a family of books written by Emily Thacker. In the same manner as other natural health books written by Emily, *The Cinnamon Book* delves into the many uses for cinnamon, both as a natural health remedy and around the home.

(For additional information on the other home health remedy and cleaning books, such as vinegar, honey, garlic, baking soda and hydrogen peroxide, please refer to the back of this book. There, you will find a description of each of these books, and many more. All of these amazing books contains hundreds of home remedies, natural cleaning solutions and recipes to simplify life and make for better well-being.)

You already know it is good for you, you just never knew HOW good it was! Or, how much cinnamon to take, or when to take it, or what kind is best…the list goes on and on. These questions might seem overwhelming, but we promise to make it simple.

And with drug prices skyrocketing and our healthcare system becoming ever more unstable, more and more people every day are turning to alternative options for healthcare than ever before. They are looking for natural alternatives in place of traditional medications as a way of taking the reins and putting healthcare back into their own hands. Too often we find ourselves reaching for the latest fad drug or heavily promoted medication instead of first looking to what nature has to offer as a safe alternative. Drug store medications are not only pricey, but often times come with unpleasant side effects which can seem as bad or worse than the treatment they were taken for in the first place.

And have you ever considered what would happen if there were a shortage of medication in the drug stores? Or, if something made it impossible to get to those stores? What about an epidemic outbreak? Drugs are all but guaranteed to be in short supply during these times of panic.

So, are we saying to stop taking pharmaceutical medications altogether? Absolutely not. But you may find this book useful as a guide to begin a conversation with your own personal healthcare provider about alternative ways to deal with some conditions or illnesses. And, it may be beneficial to look into the healing properties of cinnamon as a preventative measure to incorporate into your health care routine to stave off future problems. It is always better to prevent an illness, than to try and cure it.

At this point, you may be asking yourself these questions:

- What is so special about cinnamon?

- What makes cinnamon different than other spices?

- An entire book about cinnamon? Really?

- What does cinnamon have to offer ME?

Cinnamon is known to be a very unique spice in regard to its chemical makeup and natural healing properties. Unlike many spices, cinnamon has been found to contain curative properties unique to itself. Generations have sworn by its effectiveness and have long passed down natural health remedies for a multitude of conditions and ailments. Some with amazing results.

The fact is, there is so much information about the topic of cinnamon we are hard pressed to cover it in a single book! Healing properties, historical and folk uses, aromatherapy, research studies and trials, recipes and concoctions are just the beginning of cinnamon's amazing story.

So where do we start? Let's begin with what we know about cinnamon.

Cinnamon is an amazing spice with some of the most interesting qualities and characteristics of any of our home remedy foods. And, it's everywhere.

Spice up your life with the taste of fantastic cinnamon.
It is the star of the spice world! Cinnamon shows up in everything from coffee and tea to meats and vegetables and is irreplaceable in many desserts. Its fragrance is unmistakable; its aroma calming and pleasant.

On the pages that follow you will find just a hint of the many healthy, delicious ways to use cinnamon in the kitchen and around the home.

You have probably read magazine articles on the uses of cinnamon before. Or maybe have countless recipes of your own in which cinnamon is used to spice up the flavor of a favorite bread or cookie. Cinnamon has been long used world-wide, nearly since the beginning of time, as a wonderful accompaniment to an assortment of dishes.

Cinnamon is a common cooking spice in the Mediterranean and throughout the world. In France, for example, cinnamon is commonly used to bring out the flavor of sweet dishes. Mexican culture is proud to claim cinnamon in a vast array of recipes, from bean and rice dishes to delicious breads and desserts. Turkey, on the other hand, is known for using cinnamon to enhance savory cuisine.

This versatile spice is also a holiday staple. Not only does it sell in record amounts to be used in Thanksgiving desserts and cookies at Christmas time, but its distinctive aroma can be counted on to bring festive joy to each memorable celebration.

But more recently, cinnamon has made headlines for a very different reason. Research is backing up what our grandparents and great grandparents have known for generations: that cinnamon has amazing medicinal properties that may actually go well beyond its use in soothing an upset stomach or stopping the pain of an aching tooth.

It is with this fact in mind that *The Cinnamon Book* was written. Besides being one of the more delicious and aromatic spices Americans are familiar with, cinnamon naturally contains a wealth of medicinal properties making it extremely effective in natural home health remedies. Research studies prove that cinnamon is found to contain many necessary attributes for healing the human body.

Some of these qualities may come as a surprise to you. As you will read in greater detail later in this book, it contains properties as an:

- Antioxidant

- Antiseptic

- Anti-clotting source

- Anti-inflammatory agent

- Anti-tumor properties

- Antibacterial

- Anti-parasitic

- Antimicrobial

- Antifungal

- Immunomodulatory regulator

You will also find information on:

- The latest research studies

- What's on the horizon

Ready for another fact you may not have known about cinnamon?

Did you know most "cinnamon" purchased in the United States is not true cinnamon at all? It is a little known fact that American cinnamon is actually a cousin to the true form of cinnamon found overseas. So, does the cinnamon spice found here still contain all the amazing natural healing properties of truer cinnamons grown overseas? The answer is usually "yes." But this book will tell you exactly what to look for when purchasing cinnamon, and what the differences are in its various types.

We will also learn about several precautions that should always be taken when adding cinnamon to any diet for healing purposes, including interactions with other drugs or medical conditions to be on alert for.

We'll also discuss the very latest in research studies concerning cinnamon's most promising healing properties. Find out what direction the newest research is going and how it directly affects people suffering from diabetes, heart conditions, memory ailments such as Alzheimer's or dementia and other conditions. Many of these new studies are showing favorable results in easing symptoms of these diseases, and in some cases, preventing or curing them altogether.

When one thinks of cinnamon, we tend to think of either the ground powdery substance we measure out for recipes or perhaps thoughts of nostalgic cinnamon sticks poking out of a warm cup of tea or apple cider. *The Cinnamon Book* covers the various available forms of cinnamon and what the pros and cons are for each one. You will read about what the differences are in these various forms of cinnamon and where to purchase them. We will discuss each form, what to expect in regard to shelf life, and the best, most effective way to use each one, so you can get the most from your cinnamon experience.

We will also delve into the research behind using cinnamon as a weight loss aid, and what we can realistically expect to achieve from its use. Read about the much heralded Cinnamon Diet and what it might offer you.

And, we have also included a Frequently Asked Question section that can be used as a quick reference guide for all your most pressing cinnamon questions. In it, you'll be reminded of:

- Which type of cinnamon works best for specific uses

- The best way to store cinnamon for longer shelf life

- Where to purchase cinnamon in bulk

- Warnings and cautions for using cinnamon and what to watch out for

- ...and much more.

And while *The Cinnamon Book* was intentionally written with its use as a natural healing element in mind, no publication on cinnamon could be complete without recipes. In fact, *The Cinnamon Book* contains some of the most scrumptious recipes ever, all showcasing this amazing spice. This will help make it easier to incorporate cinnamon into your daily diet in a fun, delicious way! There are even recipes located throughout the Best Cinnamon Recipes Ever chapter to enjoy the healing effects of cinnamon with low-fat and heart healthy recipes.

What would a recipe section on cinnamon be without mentioning cinnamon buns? That all-time favorite cinnamon treat! As an added bonus, we have dedicated an entire chapter to the cinnamon bun and spin-off recipes for you to enjoy!

We genuinely hope this book will serve as useful to your family on introducing cinnamon as a natural healing agent. Be sure to share with Emily your own healing remedies as you discover hundreds of ways to incorporate this amazing spice into your everyday world. Sharing these remedies and recipes are an excellent way to ensure the tradition of using cinnamon for better health will be passed on to the next generation.

So, pour yourself a cup of hot tea, splash in that cinnamon stick and let's explore *The Cinnamon Book* together!

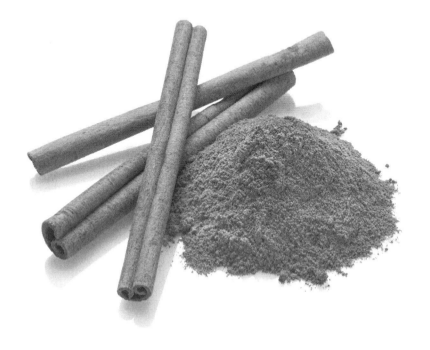

CHAPTER TWO
The History of Cinnamon

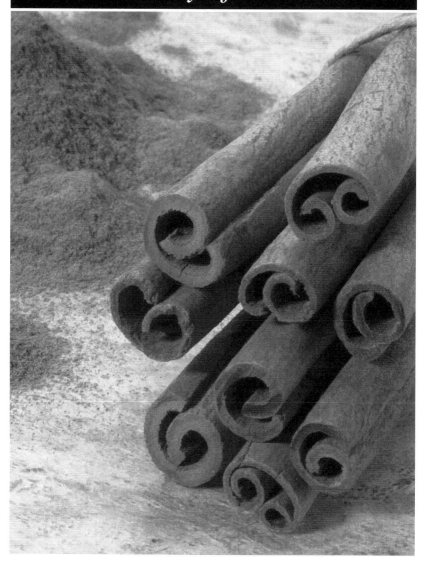

Cinnamon in time

Cinnamon has been used as a spicy seasoning for at least 5,000 years. As one of the earliest known spices it was, at times, worth more than its weight in gold! Wars were fought for control of its trade and the secrets of its production. Due to its high value, at times it was diluted with sugar, ground walnut shells or ginger roots to extend its volume and make it go farther possible to increase profits.

Cinnamon was so highly regarded in ancient times that it was considered to be a gift fit for rulers and deities. The Bible mentions cinnamon as being used for anointing, consecrating and as an aromatic perfume. The Egyptians used it for embalming purposes, and many civilizations depended on cinnamon as an anointing or cleansing oil.

- The Romans believed the cinnamon spice was sacred, and treated it as such.

- It has been said that Queen Cleopatra of Egypt used aromatic cinnamon oil as one of her most seductive love potions.

Because of the great value of cinnamon as a spice, those who traded in it worked very hard at keeping its origins a secret. Complicated stories were made up to both enhance its magical properties and to cloak its origins, allowing its value to remain nearly priceless. A few of these long, mythical tales include:

- Out at the edge of the world, at the very source of the great river Nile, cinnamon could be found, where it was fished up in huge nets.

- Another tale is told of the great phoenix of mythical fame, when faced with old age climbed into a nest of cinnamon sticks, which it then set on fire. The bird was consumed in this funeral pyre. From the ashes of that cinnamon infused nest, a new phoenix arose with the morning sun. Some believe this myth is a metaphor for Christ's resurrection.

- Giant flying creatures, the cinnamon birds, collected sticks from far off, unknown lands, and used them to build their nests. Then, harvesters came in and offered the birds huge chunks of meat. The greedy birds would carry so much meat to their nests that they would collapse from the weight. Then, at great peril to the laborers, the cinnamon sticks were gathered.

It would be near the end of the Middle Ages before the Western world learned that cinnamon was actually produced from the branches of small trees that grew throughout the Eastern world.

This knowledge helped to encourage the Europeans to look for shorter, easier routes to Asia, thereby launching an age of great discovery and exploration. Cinnamon's place as an important spice did not begin to decline until it was faced with stiff competition for the Western palate by newly discovered coffees, teas, sugars and luscious chocolates.

Expensive commodity

Throughout history, cinnamon's value was appreciated. Because cinnamon was native to East Asia and India, countries went to great lengths to bring the spice to their own home countries. People of West Asia, Africa and Europe imported cinnamon and paid great prices to do so. The impact was not only economic, but there was also a personal cost evidenced by the bloody wars over its possession.

The reasons for this fascination with cinnamon were its obvious deliciousness in culinary applications, as well as the spice's health benefits and preservation properties. People soon realized that not only was cinnamon a flavorful addition to cooked meals, but also worked to keep food from spoiling.

The events of the Crusades spread the love of cinnamon throughout the world. Cultures from all over, including the Egyptians and Greeks and even the Abbasid and Roman Empires paid small fortunes to bring cinnamon to their doorstep.

Discovering cinnamon

No one can be truly certain of the actual date or circumstances of cinnamon's discovery. It was found in the writings of Pliny the Elder that 350 grams of cinnamon was equal in value to over five kilograms of actual silver. That means, by weight, cinnamon was worth about 15 times as much as silver. In fact at one time in history, cinnamon was actually thought to be of more valuable than gold!

Cinnamon is mentioned several times in the Bible. In Biblical times, it was mixed with other ingredients and used as an anointing oil. It was also given as a treasured gift.

We do know that cinnamon use dates back to 2800s BC, as mention was made in early Chinese writings.

It is said that after Nero ordered his wife murdered, he asked that a year's supply of cinnamon be burned as sign of his sorrow and remorse.

Throughout history, bloody wars were fought in an attempt to gain control of the cinnamon trade. All this resulted in high value and demand throughout the world. It was coveted not only due to its unique flavoring as a spice, but also its unique quality in preserving food. Its delightful aroma also helped cover up the stench of aging meats. And, cinnamon was already beginning to be used for antiseptic and curative purposes.

Cinnamon was originally only native to the island we now call Sri Lanka. (Previously, Ceylon was the name of cinnamon's country of origin.) However, by around the early 1800s, other countries began growing cinnamon trees and harvesting it themselves. This ended the monopoly Sri Lanka had on the cinnamon industry, and opened up the growth of the spice to countries such as Guyana, Java and others. Asia became a plentiful producer of cinnamon. Soon, cinnamon made its way to South America and other tropical climates, too.

As cinnamon made its way around the globe, true, native cinnamon became intermingled in trade with another type of cinnamon, that actually turned out not to be a true cinnamon at all.

How cinnamon grows

True cinnamon is a light colored, fairly sweet, mild, aromatic spice. The most widely type of what we call cinnamon is the darker, more robustly flavored cassia, or sweet wood cinnamon. This is the cinnamon that almost all scientific testing has been done on, the cinnamon that you are most likely to find ground up on your grocery store shelves. Both are good for cooking and may be used interchangeably in recipes.

If left to grow wild, cinnamon would become a small evergreen tree. When cultivated, it is kept cut back to form a tall shrub by coppicing it after about two years of growth. This is accomplished by cutting the trunk of the tree off near ground level. Shoots spring up all around the newly cropped tree trunk, supplying the straight branches needed for cinnamon production. Each shrub-sized tree will form about a dozen new shoots. The tree is kept cut back so that the continuously forming new branches do not reach more than ten feet into the air.

Today, especially in Indonesia, cinnamon is often used in developing sustainable coffee plantations. By interplanting this tree turned into a shrub with coffee plants the cinnamon supplies the shade small coffee plants require and at the same time, provides a cash crop during the non-productive years while the coffee plant matures.

Harvesting cinnamon

Traditionally, cinnamon has been harvested by cutting off its long branches, beating them with a hammer in order to loosen the inner bark, then peeling the inner bark loose from the both the core and the outer bark. These strips immediately curl themselves into long rolls, called quills. This must be done as soon as the branches are cut. Once dry, the quills are cut into two to four inch lengths for shipping. Recently, mechanical harvesting devices are beginning to replace the traditional, more labor intensive manner of harvesting cinnamon

The fight for cinnamon

As previously mentioned, cinnamon was such a popular and coveted spice, that countries went to war over its trade. It was said that he who controlled the island of Ceylon, controlled its cinnamon.

History indicates that around the early 1600s, the Portuguese army landed on the island of Ceylon and took control of the cinnamon trade for Portugal. From then on, and for many centuries, wars were conducted to gain control of cinnamons fertile growing ground. Control of the island changed hands countless times. The Portuguese, French, Dutch and English all took turns conquering the island and staking claim to its trade.

Eventually, starter plants were taken from cinnamon's native island and transported to other parts of the world. Soon the growing and harvesting of cinnamon began to expand. Most of these new, cinnamon-producing countries were in tropical locations that were conducive to cinnamon's growing needs and mimicking its native homeland.

Newly planted cinnamon groves began showing up all around the world. The trees thrived in countries like Indonesia, South American countries and islands throughout the Pacific.

As cinnamon began being harvested from many countries around the world, its price eventually dropped and it became available to the masses. No longer was cinnamon the rarity once believed to have been magically fished out of the Nile river. Hence, cinnamon became even more widely used than ever before. It became more and more popular and affordable throughout the world.

With such a rich yet bloody history, one might wonder what was so worth the cost. Cinnamon was being found to have more and more uses than once thought and new discoveries putting this spice to work in a multitude of settings was happening more and more often. While originally cinnamon was perceived as the ultimate culinary spice for both its flavor and its food preservation qualities, focus began to shift from culinary delights to medicinal properties.

Use in Traditional Medicine

There is much wisdom embedded in old-time remedies. More and more, medical research confirms the value of remedies our ancestors used instinctively. These old remedies soothe the discomfort of many chronic conditions and can bring relief from troubling maladies. Some of the very best potions, nostrums and advice of long ago recognized the healing properties of cinnamon. A few are more folklore than fact; some are more fun than useful; others are of immeasurable help. Folklore or fact, fun, useful or helpful, it is for you, the reader, to decide.

- In addition to the relaxing effect of this sweet, delicious spice many have long held the belief that cinnamon will cure many diseases.

- Some civilizations looked to cinnamon as an aphrodisiac.

- Want to get going? Have more energy? Traditionally, cinnamon has been considered to be an invigorating spice, capable of energizing both the body and spirit.

- In Medieval times cinnamon was used to treat coughs and hoarseness, sore throats and colds.

Once the Crusaders brought cinnamon home with them, its use exploded. The spice was important for flavoring foods, but was also the spice of choice for concocting amorous love potions and perfumes.

That means, by weight, cinnamon was worth about 15 times as much as silver.

Cinnamon has been used since the earliest of times to help the body kill invading bacteria and viruses. It has been said to work by strengthening the immune system and invigorating the body's natural healing abilities. As more and more knowledge of cinnamon's healthy properties emerged, its use as a medicinal aid grew and physicians and families alike swore by the cinnamon spice to treat illnesses.

Prior to the discovery of antibiotics, cinnamon was used as a treatment for numerous infections and illnesses. It was applied directly to the skin, administered orally, and even inhaled for diseases such as tuberculosis.

Cinnamon's rich and fascinating history as an effective healing agent made it a valuable addition to the world of natural home remedies.

CHAPTER THREE
What is Cinnamon?

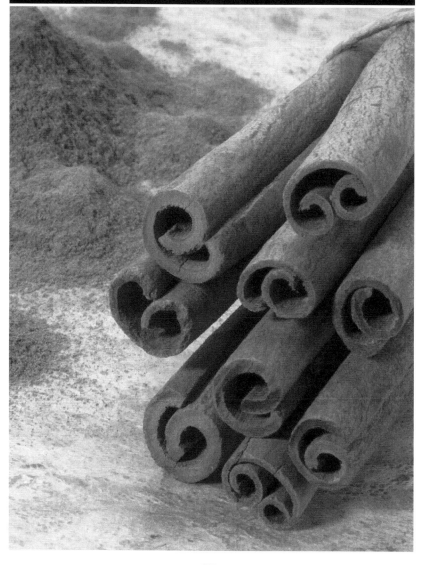

So, we know countries fought to the death over the cinnamon trade, and believed it was the answer for so many ailments and physical conditions. But what is cinnamon?

Sure, we all know cinnamon to be that wonderful spice incorporated into your grandmother's old-fashioned raisin bread or stirred into a favorite cup of warm tea. And what about the world famous cinnamon bun? Don't most of us associate that unmistakable aroma of fresh cinnamon sticks with cherished Christmas time celebrations?

But what exactly IS cinnamon? What makes it different than every other spice? And what is there about it that makes it so effective as a natural home health remedy for countless ailments and health maladies spanning generations of use?

Cinnamon, in its truest form, is a spice that is harvested from the inner bark of the cinnamon tree. While this hardy tree is native to Sri Lanka, which produces almost 90% of the world's cinnamon, it can also now be found in several Asian countries, such as Brazil, India and China.

When the cinnamon tree reaches maturity, care is taken to strip the tree of its outer bark. It is the tree's inner bark where cinnamon can be found. The inner bark of the tree is then beaten to loosen its holding, and scraped out of the tree into meter long rolls. These rolls are then permitted to dry. It is through the drying process that allows the bark to curl into the familiar "scroll" shape associated with cinnamon sticks. Next, they are cut into manageable size sticks of 2 – 4 inches, packaged for sale, and shipped around the world. For ground cinnamon, dried cinnamon sticks are pulverized into a fine powder and sold under various brand names.

Some harvesters of cinnamon have been known to treat cinnamon bark with a chemical solution during its drying period as a way of combating insects or infestation. While most reputable harvesters steer clear of this practice, it should be known that pretreating the drying bark can have negative effects on its ultimate quality. There is such a thing as "organic" cinnamon. Organic cinnamon is usually guaranteed free of any pesticides or additives.

Ceylon and Cassia: Two types of cinnamon

Throughout the world, there are more than 100 varieties or types of cinnamon. However, in the United States of America, we primarily have only two cinnamons. Believe it or not, the cinnamon we use around our home and in our favorite delectable recipes usually isn't even true cinnamon!

Cinnamon is generally divided up into two groups of either cassia or Ceylon cinnamon. While many times these names are used interchangeable, in reality they are two very different cinnamons.

While both Ceylon and cassia cinnamon possess many of the same characteristics, the only "true" cinnamon is considered to be Ceylon cinnamon. Ceylon cinnamon is taken directly from the Cinnamomum zeylanicum plant. Its name in fact, means "true cinnamon." Its sticks are lighter in color than the more familiar cassia, and the sticks tend to be dense, as opposed to open tubing thru the centers. Ceylon is also more expensive than its counterfeit cousin, with a slightly milder taste.

Cassia, on the other hand, has a darker bark and houses the infamous "scroll" shape we associate with cinnamon sticks. It is more potent in its flavoring that Ceylon and less expensive. Most cinnamon sticks purchased in American stores are of this variety.

One of the most notable differences between the two cinnamons, and a difference that is particularly important when using cinnamon for natural home remedy purposes, is its chemical make up. While both cinnamons can be used interchangeably with little or no noticeable difference in most cooking and baking applications, these differences become somewhat more apparent when used as a medicinal tool.

Coumarin is a chemical compound found in both varieties of cinnamon. This compound is a known anti-coagulant. True Ceylon cinnamon contains a negligible 0.4% coumarin compared to a full 5% coumarin in cassia. While this comparison makes no difference to the health of most people, there is a percentage of the population struggling with conditions which may be affected by increased coumarin levels. As with beginning any new routine, your personal health care practitioner should be consulted before beginning any health care regimen to ensure you are not one of the people affected by coumarin. People who have been told to eliminate or beware of coumarin levels in their diet for health reasons should be cautious of adding too much cassia cinnamon to their diets.

The part where this gets tricky is how to tell the difference between the two types of cinnamon when purchasing. The Food and Drug Administration (FDA) does not require manufacturers in the United States to divulge which type of cinnamon is being purchased. Looking on the label may be of no help.

While the FDA does not require ingredient labeling of either Ceylon or cassia cinnamon, there are a few ways to visually inspect the varieties prior to purchasing. Below is a handy chart which lists some of the more pronounced differences between the two types of cinnamon. Many of these differences can be noted by comparing the two cinnamons side by side.

	Ceylon	Cassia
Color	Pale, tan, light color	Deep red, rich color
Aroma	Lightly fragrant	Potent fragrance
Taste	Lighter sweet flavor	Stronger taste
Texture	Less firm	More firm
Cost	More expensive	Less expensive
Stick	Dense centers, thin layers	More tubular, hollow, scrolls
Coumarin	.04% coumarin	5% coumarin

For users interested in purchasing the Ceylon variety of cinnamon, there are many manufacturers which sell this product. For references on where to purchase Ceylon cinnamon, see the Frequently Asked Question section in the back of this book. There, you will find several suggestions on how to purchase Ceylon cinnamon. In addition, cinnamon capsules can be purchased at many health food or nutrition stores, and through the Internet. Again, be sure to check into which type of cinnamon was used to manufacture the capsules. With more health conscious Americans turning to cinnamon, some of the Ceylon variety capsules in health stores are marked as such.

Are there health benefits to the cassia variety?

With all the talk about the excellent benefits of the more expensive Ceylon cinnamon, one begins to wonder if the more commonly found variety of cassia cinnamon still offers medicinal benefit. The answer more times than not is YES!

Researchers have gone back and forth as to which type of cinnamon is actually better for health, but the final verdict is still out. Cassia cinnamon has much of the same make up and similarities as Ceylon, making it very useful for natural health.

While the cassia variety does contain more coumarin than the Ceylon variety, unless high quantities are taken this is still usually considered safe for people who do not have issues with coumarin. Some researchers even believe cassia cinnamon may do a better job in stabilizing glucose levels than Ceylon.

The fact is, some health experts claim Ceylon cinnamon is the better of the two, and equally, other health experts tout the benefits of cassia cinnamon.

In order to make your own choice, it's good to understand both sides of the argument. Ceylon cinnamon does contain lesser amounts of coumarin for those who find it necessary to watch its intake. Studies have been found indicating both types work well to regulate blood sugar levels. Many people base their decision on taste preference and cost considerations.

Forms of cinnamon

Like most people, when you heard the word "cinnamon" your mind probably fixated on either the ground, powdery spice we commonly use in recipes, or perhaps the cinnamon stick we use to flavor a favorite tea or hot cocoa. Just like its multitude of uses, cinnamon is equally generous in the variety of forms for which it is available.

So, which form of cinnamon is best used for what circumstance? Let's take a look and take some of the mystery out of a few of the most common (and not so common) forms of cinnamon:

- **Cinnamon sticks.** Also called quill, or cinnamon bark as it is sometimes referred to, is the inner bark of the Asian cinnamon tree which has been scraped from the tree, and allowed to dry into its familiar scroll shape. Cinnamon sticks are most often used for flavoring warm beverages, such as teas and coffees. They can also be used for flavoring sauces and stews, as the sticks are then removed prior to serving.

  The wonderful aroma of cinnamon sticks also lends them to amazing potpourris, as well as holiday decorations and centerpieces.

Cinnamon bark is one of the few spices than can even be eaten directly, if you wish to.

As a rule of thumb, cinnamon sticks tend to be a bit expensive, especially when compared to the ground or powdered version of the spice. One question that often arises when mentioning the use of cinnamon sticks is whether they must be discarded after each use, or whether they can be reused. This is a great question and has an equally great answer! Cinnamon sticks CAN be reused!

To reuse cinnamon sticks, be sure to remove them from any liquid they have been submersed or drenched in, and allow the stick to dry completely. Then wrap them tightly and save them for use another day!

It should be noted that cinnamon sticks that have been chewed on or otherwise come in contact with non-sterile applications should not be reused, as bacteria may have a chance to grow.

- **Ground cinnamon.** Also called cinnamon powder. This powder has been ground or finely grated from the dried bark of the cinnamon tree. This is the most popular form of cinnamon sold in supermarkets today, and is mainly used as a spice in cooking and baking recipes or as a flavoring condiment. In the United States, cinnamon is often used in sweet dishes, while the spice is mainly used in savory dishes in the Mideast.

- **Cinnamon oil.** Cinnamon oil is oil that is distilled out of either the leaf or bark of the cinnamon tree, and is generally amber in color. While oil obtained from the bark of the tree is somewhat stronger in nature than that from the leaf and highly concentrated, both types tend to be very caustic if handled undiluted. Great care should be taken to dilute the oil within another substance, such as water or alcohol. The oil form of cinnamon should not be consumed on a long-term daily basis. Many people believe that although bark oil is stronger than leaf oil, both can be used interchangeably in home health remedies.

  Cinnamon leaf oil. May possess an aroma more like cloves. Leaf oil tends to be the stronger of the two oils. Has also been found to kill mosquito larvae in research testing.

  Cinnamon bark oil. Aroma derived from bark tends to smell like the more familiar spice. Oil obtained from tree bark, while still potent, is slightly weaker in intensity than that of leaf oil.

- **Cinnamon extract.** Cinnamon extract is a diluted, water-soluble version of cinnamon oil. Cinnamon extract is one-fourth as potent as cinnamon oil, making it less concentrated and an ideal choice for flavorings in cooking and baking recipes. Although somewhat diluted from cinnamon oil, cinnamon extract can still be helpful in maintaining healthy living.

- **Cinnamon capsules.** Cinnamon capsules are prepackaged and sold in many health and general nutrition stores. They are often taken to aid in weight loss along with a variety of other conditions. If coumadin levels are a concern, care should be taken to purchase the Ceylon variety of cinnamon capsules, and may be listed in the ingredient list on the bottle. For general purposes, one 2,000 mg dose in cinnamon capsules is equivalent to about 1/2 to 3/4 teaspoon of ground cinnamon.

- **Cinnamon tablets.** Cinnamon tablets are identical to prepackaged cinnamon capsules and are also sold in health and nutrition stores. As with capsules, if coumadin levels are a concern, care should be taken to purchase the Ceylon variety of cinnamon capsules, and may be listed in the ingredient list on the bottle.

- **Cinnamon tincture.** Cinnamon tincture is produced in the same manner as any other tincture. A tincture is a highly concentrated extract in which an herb or spice is immersed in alcohol. For a cinnamon tincture, about 10 tablespoons of ground cinnamon are combined with one and a fourth cup of alcohol, such as Vodka.

This tincture can then be added to drinks such as coffees or teas, or incorporated into other remedies. It is said to be useful in treating indigestion, improving circulation, and easing the effects of the cold or flu.

Where to purchase

Cinnamon is one of the most common spices on grocer's shelves today and is in ample supply at most stores. Depending on what type of cinnamon you wish to purchase, and in what form, there are manly cost-effective places to begin your search.

For the ever popular ground or powdered cinnamon, you will be able to find cinnamon on the spice rack in grocery stores in ample supply. Most of these packages are small in size, containing 1 oz. to 3-4 oz. of cinnamon. This may be a good choice as you begin to investigate whether cinnamon home remedies are right for you.

As your need for cinnamon grows, however, you may want to consider purchasing cinnamon in bulk. Packages containing 20 ounces or more of cinnamon are commonly found online, in health food stores, and can even be purchased by speaking with your grocer's manager directly. Cinnamon purchased in bulk is significantly less expensive than buying the smaller, more common packages. Buying cinnamon in bulk can save both time and energy, and allow you the freedom of incorporating the spice into your daily recipes and regimen more freely and without worry of running out.

If your wish is to purchase the Ceylon variety of cinnamon, you will need to be more deliberate in your approach. As stated earlier, the exact type of cinnamon is not required to be noted on packaging labels in the United States. You may wish to consult the list showing the differences in Ceylon and cassia cinnamons to determine which cinnamon is being sold. You may also have better luck purchasing the Ceylon variety at a health food or nutrition store, although one could expect to pay more money there. Try looking online at various health shops for Ceylon cinnamon. There are some excellent deals through the Internet, and much of the Ceylon variety is sold in bulk (for greater savings), and various forms such as capsules and tablets.

Cinnamon sticks can also be readily found at your favorite grocery store. Many times both varieties are sold, making it easy to tell the difference by visual inspection.

Cinnamon extracts are sometimes sold in the spice section of your grocery store, alongside other flavorings like vanilla extract. Many times it is easier to find cinnamon extract around the holidays, as store sometimes carry this as a seasonal item. It can also be readily purchased online, or at many gourmet baking shops.

Try looking for cinnamon oil at gourmet baking shops where one might purchase flavorings for candy making. You should also be able to find it at some health food or nutrition stores. And, like the extract version, cinnamon oil can always be found online.

Cinnamon tablets and capsules are most readily available at health food and nutrition stores, although more and more drug sections of grocery stores are beginning to carry them. Competitive prices may also be found online.

Lesser known organic cinnamons can again be found at some health food or nutrition stores, organic food shops or, in greater supply, through online retailers.

Simple Storage

Now that you have made the decision as to which type and form of cinnamon is best for you, the next step is preserving that purchase as long as possible.

As with most spices, cinnamon, both ground or stick variety, is best stored in a tightly sealed container in a cool, dry place. Cinnamon extracts and oils can be stored in their original bottle, in any cool location away from direct sunlight. Tablets and capsules can be stored in the same location you would store vitamin tablets, in a cabinet away from direct heat or sunlight. None of these need to be refrigerated, although I know some people who swear by refrigerating or even freezing ground cinnamon or sticks (NOT the extract or oil) to extend shelf life.

While many chefs suggest rotating spices every 6 to 12 months, the truth is the shelf life of cinnamon (and most spices) is much greater. Spices do not tend to "go bad" anyway, or make users sick after the expiration date. They just tend to lose some of their potency in flavor after long periods of time. With the expense associated with spices, maybe some common sense is called for.

However, a more realistic approach to the longevity of spices is widely agreed upon:

Spice	Shelf life
Ground or powdered spices (cinnamon)	3 years
Herb-based spices (thyme, basil, etc.)	2 years
Cinnamon extract	4-5 years
Cinnamon oil	4-5 years
Cinnamon tablets	Check manufacturer's suggested expiry date
Cinnamon capsules	Check manufacturer's suggested expiry date

What to do with "old" cinnamon

So, you have been cleaning out your kitchen pantry and found an old, dusty bottle or jar of cinnamon deeply buried in the back. You are not certain when you purchased it, but are pretty sure it has been in there WAY past the recommended usage or expiration date. What should you do?

Throw it out? Don't even consider throwing old or dated cinnamon away!

First of all, like most spices, cinnamon does not "go bad." It will not deteriorate to the point of causing sickness if ingested. "Old" cinnamon merely loses a bit of its flavor over time, and some of its potency as a natural home health remedy.

If you are determined to use cinnamon within its expiration date, I have great news for you. Expired cinnamon still has a multitude of uses around the home and outdoors! In fact, even "old" cinnamon that has been found buried in an old drawer or spice rack will do just fine! It's a great way to put older, forgotten bottles of cinnamon to great use instead of throwing them out.

As a reminder, remember that the most important reasons for being conscious of the expiration or best use date on spices are due to flavor and potency. But in this chapter we are dealing with using cinnamon around the home, and out in the garden on plants and other vegetation. We are not looking to reap the same potential health results we might be looking for with natural home health remedies. In these cases, cinnamon can be used well past any expiration date written on the jar. In fact, in these circumstances, cinnamon can be used indefinitely!

And, when talking about the use of cinnamon in home or gardening applications, any type of cinnamon will work equally as well. No need to worry about purchasing the more expensive Ceylon cinnamon. ANY type of cinnamon will do the job just fine. The extra expense of Ceylon cinnamon is unwarranted and reaps no extra benefits here.

This is another wonderful reason to purchase cinnamon in bulk, buy cinnamon that is an unknown variety, or even use a few bottles of cinnamons friends or family are planning to discard. If you find that large containers of cinnamon that were purchased in bulk are reaching the expiration date, simply mark them for household use.

(Although this generally isn't necessary, as the potency and flavor effects are usually minimal enough not to make any noticeable difference).

What about other "cinnamons?"

You may have read about a few other "cinnamons" that are becoming more and more common. Talk of cinnamon trees and cinnamon plants (such as cinnamon basil) are popping up around nurseries and garden centers. So, what exactly are these plants, and are they really true cinnamon?

Cinnamon trees and cinnamon plants are not true cinnamon. However, that does not mean there is no benefit to these plants. As you will read in a later chapter, Cinnamon Around the Home, cinnamon trees and plants can often mimic some of the wonderful effects of true cinnamon, and can be of great benefit in outdoor applications.

Cinnamon tree can mean several different plants. True cinnamon trees refer to the cinnamon tree found in Sri Lanka or other countries in that part of the world. Cinnamon trees have also been imported and are growing in other areas under climate controlled greenhouses. True cinnamon trees thrive in tropical climates. "Imitation" cinnamon trees are also popping up that have been genetically altered to give the appearance of cinnamon. Some of these can be wonderful additions to garden landscapes not only for their beauty, but also as a way of keeping destructive insects at bay.

Cinnamon basil is not true cinnamon, but does have the same aromatic scent as cinnamon, along with some of its insect repelling properties. Cinnamon basil contains cinnamate, which is the chemical in real cinnamon that gives the spice its familiar flavor and aroma. Cinnamon basil can be eaten, or planted in gardens around other plants to help repel bugs and other harmful insects.

Health properties

So, what makes cinnamon so special? Why is it touted as one of the best natural remedy sources available for fighting everything from mouth sores to stomach ulcers?

A great deal of research has been conducted into the chemical composition of cinnamon, and what that make up might mean for the human body. While this research is ongoing, there is one thing we know for certain. When used properly, cinnamon can play an effect role as both a natural healing agent, as well as a preventative for many conditions, ailment and diseases.

Cinnamon contains a host of vitamin and minerals needed for healthy body function and healing. A few of those elements include manganese, zinc, calcium, iron, niacin and even potassium. Cinnamon also contains quantities of Vitamins A, C and K, as well as being naturally high in fiber.

Research into cinnamon has also proven the spice contains countless medicinal qualities which make it ideal for treating numerous health conditions. A few of these stunning attributes include:

- Antiseptic properties

- Anti-clotting effect

- Anti-inflammatory agent

- Anti-tumor properties

- Antibacterial

- Antimicrobial

- Antiparasitic

- Antifungal

- Antioxidant properties

All of these qualities work to make cinnamon an excellent choice as a natural health remedy. While we are certainly able to purchase a multitude of pharmaceutical medications with the same qualities, you will find that you would be hard pressed to find a single over the counter or prescription medication which carries ALL of the attributes in the same pill. Plus, using cinnamon may be a way to avoid many of the unwanted or even harmful medical side effects sometimes associated with these popular drugs. And, with cinnamon being readily available at every corner supermarket, and its relatively inexpensive price tag when compared with manufactured medications, cinnamon might be the medicinal answer we have all been waiting for.

Let's explore these attributes in greater depth in the next chapter, as well as finding out how to use these qualities in home remedies of your own!

CHAPTER FOUR
The Healing Properties of Cinnamon

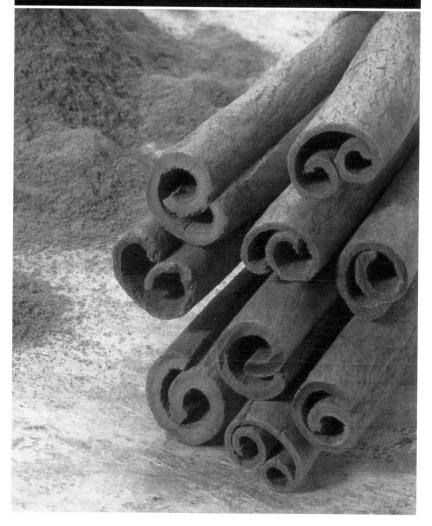

What will you do when antibiotics no longer work? What will happen when disaster strikes? Or the plague sets in?

Knowledge of what to do during an epidemic or when more traditional medicines are not available could save your life. There are things in your kitchen that can help to protect your family when there is a pandemic emergency and you are faced with:

- Swine flu

- Avian flu

- MRSA

- West Nile virus

- Staph, strep, hospital acquired infections

- Meningitis

- Diabetes

Because cinnamon is able to affect blood sugar, bacteria and fungus, it may be one of those items that stand between you and disaster. Another important feature of using foods to treat illnesses is that they do not become ineffective against germs or lead to the development of buildup drug resistant strains of germs such as often happens with prescription medicines. And, you do not have to worry about the side effects of antibiotics and other powerful drugs.

We know cinnamon improves health by being antibacterial and anti fungus. As an antibiotic, it fights helicobacter pylori, a leading cause of stomach ulcers. As a deterrent to fungus, it fights Candida and other yeast infections, such as thrush.

Scientists have confirmed that cinnamon has definite anti-inflammatory action. One fourth to one half a teaspoon of cinnamon each day is considered to be a therapeutic dose.

Cinnamon also is credited with being able to invigorate white cells, thereby boosting the immune system. Cinnamon is also a good source of manganese, fiber, iron and calcium.

Since cinnamon has the proven ability to lower blood sugar, if you take insulin or a blood sugar lowering pill, you may want to discuss with your healthcare provider the possibility of including some cinnamon in your everyday diet. It is possible you could lower the amount of expensive prescription medicine you take.

Cinnamon is considered to be an anticoagulant and as such is believed to help fight the possibility of heart attacks, blood clots and strokes.

Cinnamon is sometimes called a blood thinner. This is not exactly true. It alters the metabolism of vitamin K and depletes the body's supply of vitamin K. Because cinnamon hinders the synthesis of additional K, it inhibits blood from clotting. Its regular use could make it possible to take less of the dangerous chemical, warfarin.

Warfarin is a substance that lowers the body's ability to clot blood. Because this popular, very potent, ingredient of rat poison interferes with the ability of blood to clot, the rodent bleeds, usually internally, until it dies. Warfarin is the active chemical in the drug called coumadin. Some other names that warfarin is sold under include:

- Jantoven
- Marevan
- Lawarin
- Waran
- Warfant

Warfarin is a necessary precaution to help prevent blood clots in people who have certain implants, such as heart valves. Because cinnamon increases the action of the prescription medicine, coumadin, some think taking bit of cinnamon every day might lead to the possibility of taking a smaller daily dose of coumadin.

CAUTION: Always consult your healthcare professional before making any changes in medication or eating habits.

Coumarin is a component of most processed cinnamon. Some health agencies, especially those in Europe, have raised questions about the safely of ingesting large amounts of coumarin. It is thought that it may have some toxicity to the liver and kidneys. Although, most of the warnings suggest chemically produced coumarin is more dangerous and more likely to cause problems than the naturally occurring type found in cinnamon.

Cinnamaldehyde is the organic compound in cinnamon that gives it the distinctive flavor and aroma we all recognize. It inhibits production of nitric oxide, a strong free radical. Cinnamon also contains methyl-hydroxy-chalcone polymer.

Cinnamon can replace harmful chemicals used to create nanoparticles. Scientists have found a method that could replace nearly all of the toxic chemicals required to make gold nanoparticles.

Some cinnamon has been found that has retained much of its sweet aroma and taste for hundreds of years. Store cinnamon sticks in an airtight glass jar and keep them in a cool, dark, dry place. Ground cinnamon can be kept fresh longer if frozen. When buying cinnamon, check that it is fresh by smelling it.

Cinnamon is sometimes used in the pharmaceutical world for its ability to boost the power of other drugs. Cinnamon has been found to be helpful in relieving of painful stomach gas, diarrhea, nausea and to reduce flatulence.

Cinnamon oil is known to be a powerful germicide.

Cinnamon's Health Properties

For centuries, cinnamon has been used as a natural health remedy across the globe. Traditional Chinese medicine has long touted the benefits of cinnamon in treating a multitude of the body's ailments. Generations have sworn by the healing effects cinnamon has on the human body, whether it is disinfecting an open wound or settling an ulcerated stomach.

So what makes cinnamon such a potent healing agent?

For starters, cinnamon contains many vitamin and mineral nutrients necessary for healthy living. It contains high levels of the mineral manganese, which is essential in maintaining a healthy body's skin, bone, and in glucose tolerance. Manganese may also play an important role in the prevention of some neurological disorders such as Alzheimer's disease. Several studies have concluded that the aroma therapeutic aspects of cinnamon can actually improve cognitive function and memory issues.

Cinnamon also contains other minerals including zinc, calcium, iron and potassium. The niacin vitamin is also present along with Vitamins A, C and K. In addition, cinnamon is also considered to be high in fiber.

Antioxidant

One of cinnamon's most surprising attributes is its antioxidant properties. Did you know cinnamon contains 4 to 5 times as many antioxidants as a half cup of blueberries? These antioxidants can work in conjunction with the body's natural immune system to help slow down or prohibit the growth of cancer cells. A study conducted for the U.S. Department of Agriculture concluded that cinnamon reduced the growth of cancer cells in leukemia patients as well.

Research is also showing that a single teaspoon of cinnamon worked into our daily diet can help lower LDL ("bad") cholesterol. This is accomplished through cinnamon's ability to hold down inflammation in the lining of arteries, making the deposit of harmful cholesterol more difficult. This action is shown to prevent conditions such as atherosclerosis, or plaque build up in the arteries.

In addition to lowering LDL levels, cinnamon has also been linked to the possible prevention of type-2 diabetes. Since cinnamon has been shown in studies to help in the regulation of blood sugar levels, this is exciting news for diabetics. In the *Journal of the American Board of Family Medicine*, participants showed a positive effect in blood glucose levels after the consummation of cinnamon.

Multiple studies have also shown a reduction in blood pressure, both in systolic and diastolic pressure, in those people struggling with type-2 diabetes. These candidates were given doses of a mere 2 grams of cinnamon for three months, and showed remarkable results.

Anti-inflammatory
Cinnamon has always been associated with its anti-inflammatory attributes. One study in particular from the prestigious Copenhagen University asked participants to consume one half teaspoon of cinnamon each morning with breakfast. Participants reported lessening of arthritis pain, joint discomfort and inflammation by the study's end.

Antimicrobial
Cinnamon contains a compound called cinnamaldehyde, a chemical known for its antimicrobial properties. Cinnamaldehyde works to stop or slow the body's inflammatory process. This special agent has also proven to destroy a wide gamut of harmful bacteria, fungi and even stubborn viruses, making it an excellent illness-fighter.

Antiseptic

Cinnamon also contains properties that are conducive to antiseptic applications, such as treating open cuts or wounds, and preventing infection.

Anticlotting

The spice has also been shown to possess mild anticlotting qualities which can be of benefit to those who have adverse reactions when taking pharmaceutical blood thinners. However, great care should be taken for those who already have bleeding issues, as cinnamon could well indeed worsen the problem. (See A Gentle Word of Caution in the back of this book.)

Anti-fungal

In addition to being anti-microbial, cinnamon also has the amazing distinction of being anti-fungal. The highly concentrated cinnamon oil, in particular, but also the lesser concentrated cinnamon extract, have shown themselves to be helpful in treating fungal-type ailments such as vaginal yeast infections and thrush. Research has shown cinnamon to be extremely beneficial in the active treatment of head lice. It has also been found helpful in treating the root causes of many stomach ulcers.

These are just a few of main attributes cinnamon possesses which makes it an excellent choice for natural home health remedies. Time and time again, cinnamon has proven itself to be one of the more potent, beneficial spices when it comes to aiding he human body in fighting illness, general healing or preventative maintenance.

These amazing properties, when used in conjunction with the body's own natural defenses and immune system, can work to treat a multitude of conditions:

- Arthritis pain
- Battles migraine headaches
- Muscle pain
- Joint discomfort
- Excessive itching
- Aids in breast feeding
- Cold and flu
- Pain reliever
- Kill bacteria
- Combat tooth decay
- Fights infections
- Aids in memory loss

This is just a short list of some of the areas of health cinnamon can be beneficial. Let's move on and find out how to put cinnamon's amazing health properties to use.

CHAPTER FIVE
Cinnamon for Better Health

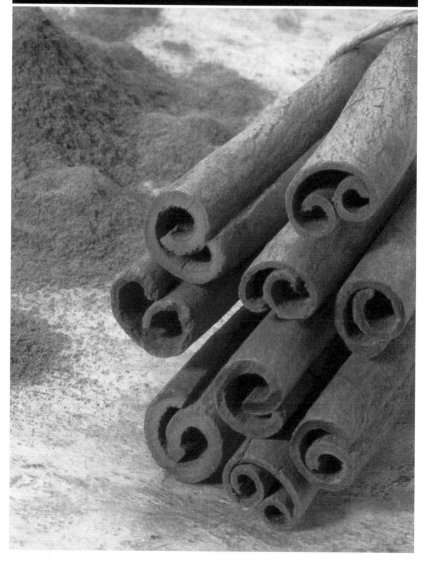

When we hear the word "cinnamon" our first thought tends to be wonderful home baked cinnamon rolls on a crisp morning, or the amazing aromatics of Christmas time. Cinnamon has seemingly endless uses in everything from hot apple cider and cinnamon bread to spicing up French toast and baked apples. But the wonderful uses for cinnamon extend much farther than just its delicious spice flavor.

The history of cinnamon dates back more than 2,700 years to the ancient orient where it can be found in archaic Chinese writings. It was a coveted spice traded between continents and even has foundations in the Bible. Cinnamon was used as not only an accompaniment for wonderful baked goods throughout the ages, but also for medicinal purposes and even as an embalming agent.

Cinnamon is even mentioned throughout the Bible. Moses was commanded to make a holy ointment as an apothecary. This ointment, containing cinnamon, was used to anoint the holy tabernacle, ark of the covenant, as well as many of the vessels throughout. Is it possible that cinnamon's healing properties were known back in Biblical times?

We do know that the history of cinnamon as a home remedy dates back thousands of years. While we know cinnamon was used mainly as a cooking spice and preservation mechanism, we also read about indications that cinnamon was used for much more.

Many believe that cinnamon was used very early on as a deterrent to illness at the first sign of infection. Cinnamon was also used as a calming aromatic to help ease tension and anxiety. And, we do know that long ago cinnamon used as a tea was used to calm aching stomachs and ease gastrointestinal issues.

Throughout the years and through much scientific research, we know that cinnamon's benefits are so much greater than we originally knew. Cinnamon is a complex spice with a multitude of health benefits.

Cinnamon's chemical make up which contains high amounts of phenol makes it a highly effective antiseptic. Today, these antiseptic uses are excellent when used as a mouthwash, for lowering blood pressure, and even preventing blood clots. Cinnamon has also been shown to work effectively in treating common colds, flu and digestive ailments. It is also rich in cancer-fighting antioxidant properties.

Many of the ailments and maladies cinnamon has been shown effective in treating include:

- Diabetes
- Cholesterol
- Heart health
- Digestive issues
- Relieves joint pain
- Arthritis
- Stimulates circulation
- Urinary tract infections
- Relieves congestion
- Stomach ulcers

- Yeast infections
- Good, preliminary evidence cinnamon may possess anticancer actions
- Dyspepsia
- Fights common cold
- Immunomodulatory properties
- Reduce proliferation of leukemia and lymphoma cancer cells
- Weight loss
- Early research is promising for use in HIV-positive patients
- Positive early studies for treatment of multiple sclerosis (MS)
- Reduces risk factors associated with heart disease
- Reduces fasting blood glucose levels.
- Fights E. coli
- Boosts memory function
- Reduce overall cholesterol
- Reduce triglyceride levels
- Reduce LDL (bad) cholesterol levels
- Lower blood sugar levels in Type 2 Diabetes
- Lower blood pressure
- Respiratory ailments
- Skin lesions and infections
- Boost brain function
- Possible cancer prevention
- Toothaches and mouth sores

Traditional medicine focuses on pharmaceuticals which can come with a heavy price tag – both financially and medically. Drug manufacturers have found their niche in a multi-billion dollar industry. The cost of medications are taking a heavier and heavier toll on the family budget, with sometimes minimal results. But the most disturbing aspect of drug medications are the bothersome, sometimes dangerous, side affects which accompany them. At times it can seem like a trade off when taking one medication, only to be troubled with an unwanted or unforeseen side effect later down the road.

Should we stop taking medications for our ailments? Not necessarily. And necessary prescriptions ordered by your health care professional can make enormous differences in our health and the way we feel. However, there are many times when one might consider trying a more natural approach to personal health care. Together, you and the partnership you have with your physician can help make the best health care decision for you. Keep the lines of communication open, and know that you do have options!

Examining natural home health remedies can offer a variety of options to you, without the high cost of manufactured drugs and medications and in most cases without harmful side effects. The benefits of 'going natural' can be enormous, and there is no better feeling in knowing you are taking charge of your own health care needs, in a safe, natural way.

Most natural health remedies have been passed down through generations, standing the test of time. So many of them can be easily adjusted to your particular need. And, after becoming more familiar with home remedies, you may even be able to adapt and provide home health remedies of your own!

In many cases we have offered specific, written out home remedies for you to try. But remember, it is okay to be flexible in your approach to natural health. Some of the easiest methods for adding cinnamon to your diet are also the most delicious. If a remedy calls for cinnamon mixed into your favorite morning coffee, for example, and you are not a coffee drinker, remember you can add cinnamon to your diet in other ways as well. Try a few of these simple ways to add a little cinnamon to your life on a daily basis for better health:

- Sprinkle a little cinnamon on top of a half a cup of applesauce

- Try a cinnamon stick swirled in a cup of warm tea

- Cinnamon on steak? Of course! In many cultures throughout the world, cinnamon is used to spice up a savory steak or other fine meats.

- Use a little cinnamon powder in your morning oatmeal

- Make a delicious spread consisting of honey and a little cinnamon to spread on a bagel or slice of toast

Try these remedies with an open mind, and see if you find yourself reaping the drug-free benefits of treating ailments, maladies and conditions without the harmful effects of so many processed drugs. Rest in the peace of mind and reassurance in the natural healing properties of cinnamon. So, before you reach for the usual drugstore medication to treat the latest ache and pain, think about giving one of these natural home remedies a try!

One word of caution. As we stated before, there is such a thing as "too much of a good thing." Like any health regimen, you should consult your health care practitioner before starting any new health care routine, cinnamon included. While there are more than one hundred types of cinnamon world wide, only two are popular in the United States. Cassia and Ceylon cinnamons are the most popular in this country, and can be found in both ground powder form and sold as a capsule. Cassia cinnamon contains higher levels of coumarin than Ceylon cinnamon, which can be dangerous in high levels for people struggling with liver disease. However, cinnamon sold in the United States is not required to divulge which type of cinnamon is being sold. Great care should be taken when adding cinnamon to a diet required to be free of coumarin. Be sure and consult your health care provider before staring any cinnamon regimen.

Lowering cholesterol

Lower cholesterol by incorporating a half teaspoon cinnamon to your daily diet. You can achieve this half teaspoon a multitude of ways.

Eat a half teaspoon of cinnamon each morning with your breakfast meal.

Mix a half teaspoon of cinnamon into your favorite coffee or tea for lower cholesterol.

Try combining cinnamon and yogurt together for an easy, cholesterol-lowering breakfast.

Another study indicates that lower cholesterol might be possible by taking either one to five grams per day of ground cinnamon, or 80 mg per day of the extract form taken as a supplement. Do NOT take both.

Not wild about cinnamon's taste, but love its cholesterol lowering effect? Try cinnamon capsules or tablets for lower cholesterol. These are pre-measured, and can be purchased at most local health food and nutrition stores.

Drink one or two cups of tea each day, say Japanese herbalists, and its phytochemicals will lower your cholesterol. This works even better with cinnamon added to the tea.

Lower cholesterol
Mix up this pleasant tasting balm and slowly sip a one third a cup of it before meals. Within two weeks cholesterol will show a significant drop.

2 tbsp honey
1 tbsp cinnamon
2 cups water

Better circulation
Sprinkle a bit of ginger and cinnamon on your food at breakfast and your blood will never get thick and fatty. Try a cup of warm cinnamon tea early in the morning to promote good circulation.

Heart health

For overall better heart health, try a paste of honey and cinnamon on bread in place of butter or jelly. It is believed to reduce cholesterol, strengthen the heart and help to prevent attacks. Many believe cinnamon restores artery flexibility and melts away clogs in aging arteries.

To keep your arteries from becoming clogged when you are old, begin when you are young to eat generous amounts of sunflower seeds, cinnamon flavored foods, sweet potatoes, cooked carrots, lentils, chicken and turkey.

Fatigue

Feeling run down and can't seem to find your stamina? Try this simple remedy. Using a small glass of water, add a teaspoon of honey with a sprinkle of ground cinnamon added to it. Drink this concoction in the morning, and repeat about mid afternoon. After about 10 days, you should begin to notice a difference in ending fatigue.

Bladder infections

Cinnamon's antiseptic qualities are ideal for treating bladder and urinary tract infections. Try this home remedy for relief.

Mix one tablespoon honey and a half teaspoon cinnamon in a glass of warm water and drink.

Congestion

Add a few drops of cinnamon oil to a warm bowl of water. Cover your head with a towel over the bowl and allow yourself to breathe in the aromatic vapor to clear a congested head.

Cough and congestion

Have a cough you can't seem to get rid of? Feeling congested? Turn to the chapter on recipes in this book and make a batch of the cinnamon glass candies or cinnamon lollipops. These cinnamon candies are a great way to add a little cinnamon to your diet and battle a nagging cough or congestion.

Colds

1 cup water
2 tsp honey
1/2 tsp cinnamon

Mix honey and cinnamon into very hot water and sip slowly to relieve the worse effects of a cold.

More cold relief

3 tbsp honey
1/3 cup cinnamon

Mix together and take a teaspoonful three times a day to clear the sinuses. This thick tonic will also cure a nagging cold in three days.

Flu

1 tbsp honey
1 tbsp cinnamon
1/2 cup water

Stir honey and cinnamon into warm water and sip throughout the day. Soon the aches and pains of flu will leave your body.

Headaches

If you drink lots of cocoa and eat oatmeal with wheat germ and cinnamon sprinkled on it you will keep headaches away.

There are several home remedies handed down through the generations to help ease headache pain. Try one of these and see which works best for you.

Slowly sip on a tea made from hot water, one tablespoon of honey and a half teaspoon of cinnamon.

Make your own poultice from cinnamon by combining a tablespoon of honey with two tablespoons of warm water. Carefully smear some of the cinnamon paste onto your forehead and relax, uninterrupted, in a dark room. You should begin to feel better in about 30 minutes.

Many people claim the fragrant aroma of cinnamon spice helps ease tension headaches. Take a large bowl of steaming hot water (being careful not to spill the water or burn yourself) and place on a table. Drop in a few drops of cinnamon oil. Sit close to the bowl and allow yourself to breathe in the cinnamon vapors to help ease headache pain.

For another aromatic approach to easing headaches, be sure and visit the section in this book entitled, Cinnamon Around the Home for a list of novel ideas illustrating how to make your own cinnamon potpourri and other concoctions to add the fragrance of cinnamon freshness around your home.

Sore throat

Try this remedy to ease an aching sore throat. Add one cinnamon stick to boiling water and allow to steep for five minutes. Remove the cinnamon stick (you can save the stick for later use!). Slowly drink a cup of this tea two or three times a day for relief from a stinging sore throat.

For a delicious way to stop an aching sore throat, make a batch of cinnamon lollipops and suck on them throughout the day. The recipe for these lollipops are in this book's chapter on Recipes.

Indigestion

Cinnamon works to block the body's natural production of inflammatory chemicals that cause inflammation and indigestion.

If you sprinkle a generous dusting of cinnamon over a tablespoon of honey and swallow it down before meals, indigestion will never cause you grief.

Steep a quarter teaspoon of cinnamon into a warm cup of water for two to three minutes. Sip on this tea for relief of indigestion.

Through the years, cinnamon has been considered an aid in the digestion of milk and dairy products. It is also considered helpful for absorbing the healthy goodness of raw fruit.

Diarrhea

An old English remedy for both dysentery and ordinary diarrhea was to sip on a cup of milk with a heaping spoonful of cinnamon stirred into it.

Gas pains

Cinnamon can reduce the amount of gas in the intestines which cause bloating pain and embarrassing situations. People of India and Japan have long used this combination of cinnamon and honey to prevent the embarrassing passage of gas.

Mix one tablespoon of honey and a half teaspoon of cinnamon in a cup of warm water and drink.

Upset stomach

Bothered by upset stomachs? Give this recipe a try for quick relief.

1 tsp honey
1/2 tsp cinnamon
1/2 cup water

Calm an upset stomach by slowly sipping water that has honey and cinnamon added to it. Do this before all meals and stomach ulcers will be relieved.

Bladder infections

Bothered by irritating bladder infections? Try this for rapid relief:

2 tbsp cinnamon
1 tsp honey
1 glass of water

Drink this mixture frequently and never be troubled by an infection of the bladder. Mixture can also be used as a preventative against reoccurring bladder infections by drinking periodically.

E. coli
Research at Kansas University show adding cinnamon to juices that are unpasteurized can help destroy dangerous E. coli bacteria.

Salmonella
Cinnamon has also been found to keep dangerous salmonella at bay in meats and other consumables.

Better brain function
Several studies have indicated that smelling cinnamon actually boosts brain and memory function. Just be careful not to sniff or inhale large quantities of cinnamon powder, as this can be irritating on the body's respiratory system.

Try adding a few drops of cinnamon oil to a bowl of hot water. Allow yourself to gently inhale the steam to help awaken memory and aid in stronger, more alert brain function.

Studies are also indicating that placing cinnamon in well traveled parts of the home may work all day long to enhance brain activity.

Tension
Boil enough water for a teacup and add a half teaspoon of cinnamon. Sit quietly in a calm room and gently sip on this tea to help bring relief to tension and worry.

Loss of hearing
Try a dose of one tablespoon of honey mixed in with a half teaspoon of cinnamon each night to help with the effects of hearing loss.

Arthritis

Suffering from arthritis pain? Cinnamon may be an answer. Cinnamon is wonderful for relieving pain associated with arthritis or stiffness in the joints as we age. Try this concoction to ease the pain.

Combine a half a teaspoon of cinnamon with one tablespoon or so of honey. You may eat this on its own, or use it as a spread over a slice of toast, bagel or English muffin. Consume this every day for three or four weeks to ease the pain of arthritis. You should begin to notice a difference after the first 10 days.

Every day, eat a salad sprinkled with olive oil, apple cider vinegar, cinnamon and garlic to stop the swelling and redness of arthritis.

For more immediate arthritis relief, simply add two to three drops of cinnamon oil to a warm compress and massage into the affected area.

1 cup water
2 tsp honey
1/2 tsp cinnamon

Mix honey and cinnamon into a cup of warm water and drink it all down before meals. Arthritis aches and pains will slowly fade away.

Try a teaspoonful of honey sprinkled with a little cinnamon each morning to help fight the pain and inflammation associated with arthritis.

More arthritis remedies

Mix three tablespoons of honey with three tablespoons of warm water. Add a half teaspoon of ground cinnamon and mix together into a gel like paste. Rub into painful arthritic joints to relieve the pain.

If ground cinnamon is unavailable, or for a slightly more potent version, use cinnamon oil in the place of ground cinnamon.

Diabetes

More and more research is beginning to indicate the effectiveness of cinnamon when dealing with the effects of diabetes.

Try consuming a half teaspoon of cinnamon each day. Over a month or so, you may see a natural decrease in blood sugar levels.

Please remember that coumarin which is found in cinnamon can also effect the body. If you are already taking medication to control or stabilize blood sugar levels, great care should be taken when considering the addition of cinnamon to your regimen. Don't forget to consult your healthcare practitioner before starting any new healthcare regimen.

Overall better health

Mix a bit of cinnamon with cloves for an extra punch of healthfulness. Cloves are an excellent combatant against nasty germs. Together, cinnamon and cloves make an excellent combination in promoting overall better health.

Bad breath

It is said that South American populations depend on cinnamon to help fight halitosis (bad breath). Just take a cup of warm water and add a teaspoon of honey and a quarter teaspoon of cinnamon. Gargle with this antiseptic solution for fresher breath as it works to kill bacteria and germs of the mouth

For a nagging sore throat, try making a batch of the cinnamon class Candies from the recipe section of this book. Pop a piece or two in your mouth and suck on the candy throughout the day to ease sore throat pain.

The recipe for cinnamon lollipops can also be found in the chapter on recipes. These are great to use throughout the day to battle an aching throat.

Combat halitosis with this simple mixture:

1 tbsp honey
1 tsp cinnamon
1 cup hot water

Mix together and drink daily.

An old time South American remedy for bad breath was to gargle each morning with a rinse of water and cinnamon.

Try brushing your teeth each morning with a little cinnamon sprinkled on your toothbrush. Gently brush up into your gums and remember to clean all areas of your tongue. Cinnamon's antibacterial qualities will work to rid your mouth of any germs that might cause unpleasant odors.

Yeast infections

As stated earlier, cinnamon has been found to possess a miraculous antifungal and antibacterial qualities which makes it ideal for treating nuisances like yeast infections. For quick relief, give this remedy a try.

Mix one cup of warm water with one tablespoon of honey and a teaspoon of cinnamon.

You can also begin with your favorite tea and add the honey and cinnamon to it.

To treat yeast infections, any type of cinnamon food will do…not just tea. Try a few cinnamon crisps or warm cinnamon toast if tea is not your thing. To find a few delicious cinnamon treats, be sure and review the chapter on recipes in the back of this book.

Insomnia

Having a difficult time falling asleep or staying asleep at night? Cinnamon and milk make a great combination to battle insomnia. Try this concoction:

1 cup of milk
1 cinnamon stick
1/2 tsp of honey

Gently warm the milk over medium heat until it is warmed throughout. Milk should be hot, but not quite to the boiling stage. Be careful not to scald or burn the milk. Pour hot milk into a glass and add one cinnamon stick, gently stirring with the stick. Allow to steep for 5 to 10 minutes. Add a half teaspoon of honey to sweeten and enjoy a better night of rest!

Hair loss

Try this recipe to stop hair loss and promote growth of new roots.

2 tbsp honey
1 tsp cinnamon
2 tbsp olive oil

Warm the olive oil in the microwave, but not too hot to the touch. Add honey and cinnamon and mix thoroughly. Rub mixture into scalp and allow to rest 10 – 15 minutes. Wash out and repeat every few days as necessary.

Skin infections

Troubled by unsightly or itching skin irritations? Give this a try to ease the symptoms of eczema and other unsightly skin infections.

1 tbsp cinnamon
1 tbsp honey

Mix together and apply to ringworm infections and areas of skin showing signs of eczema. Soon the skin will be smooth and free of ugly flaking.

Aging

Fight the effects of aging by sipping of this powerful youth promoting tonic. You will live longer and stay youthful for all of your life.

3 tbsp honey
1 tsp cinnamon
1 glass water

Cleaning cuts and wounds

To clean and disinfect a cut, wound or scrape, steep one cinnamon stick in a cup of hot water for about ten minutes. Once the water has cooled to a safe, warm temperature, use this antiseptic to clean a new cut or wound.

Did you scrape yourself outdoors and are unable to mix the water and cinnamon mixture? Not to worry. Many people sprinkle a little cinnamon directly on an open cut or scrape as a disinfectant.

A clean poultice can also be made by adding a teaspoon or so into a cup of boiling water. Allow the water to cool to a warm temperature and place a clean cloth to soak in the cinnamon water solution. Use this poultice to wrap around cut or bruised areas of the arms and legs for relief and healing.

Healthy immune system

Research indicates that cinnamon in conjunction with honey can help boost the immune system. Cinnamon's many unique properties such as being an antioxidant, antibacterial and antiseptic work together to strengthen and protect the human body.

Include cinnamon in your diet through various cinnamon dishes, teas and desserts. You can also make this wonderful spread to enjoy.

1 tbsp honey
1/4 tsp cinnamon

Mix together and enjoy on warm bagels, toast or a favorite cinnamon bread.

Weight loss

Cinnamon is renown for its ability to promote healthy weight loss. About 20 minutes before eating breakfast, drink a small glass of hot water (about 8 ounces) mixed with a tablespoon of honey and a half teaspoon of cinnamon.

Cinnamon is also effective at stopping fat build ups in the blood stream with can result in unwanted weight gain. Be sure and enjoy cinnamon throughout the day to help limit fat and cholesterol build up. You can find countless recipes in the recipe section of this book for delicious, nutritious ways to enjoy the taste and weight loss benefits of cinnamon.

Also, do not forget to consult the weight loss chapter in this book entitled, Cinnamon for Weight Loss. In it you will not only read about the science behind cinnamon's unique benefit to weight loss, but also find specific recipes geared toward this goal.

Toothaches

1 tsp cinnamon
1/4 cup honey

Stir cinnamon and honey together and dab onto an aching tooth several times a day. You will soon be free of your tooth pain.

Don't like the taste of honey? A thick dab of cinnamon can be applied directly to an aching tooth or gum area to stop the pain.

Hives

Steep one cinnamon stick in a cup of hot water for about ten minutes. Once the water has cooled to a safe, warm temperature, rinse affected area with cinnamon water to alleviate itching.

A warm cinnamon poultice can also be made by soaking a clean cloth in warm cinnamon water and wrapping the affected area.

Insect bites and bee stings

Cinnamon's antiseptic qualities are perfect to clean insect bites or stings. Simply steep one cinnamon stick in a cup of hot water for about ten minutes. Once the water has cooled to a safe, warm temperature, treat the insect bite or sting with a poultice using a clean cloth and cinnamon water. Not only will this help disinfect the bite, but it will also help treat itching associated with stings and bites.

Sore leg muscles

Sore leg muscles and cramping can be relieved with this great home remedy featuring cinnamon.

1/2 cup olive oil
1 tbsp cinnamon
1 tbsp ginger root

Rub sore leg muscles with a mixture of olive oil, cinnamon and finely minced ginger root to comfort them. This is also a good liniment for bad bruises.

Drinking water
   3 tsp cinnamon
   2 tbsp honey
   1 glass water

When worried about the healthfulness of drinking water, mix cinnamon and honey into a glass of it. Germs and bugs will be less likely to dwell in it.

Depression and the Winter Blues
   Let the effects of cinnamon revitalize you by beginning the day with a warm cup of cinnamon tea.

For more noticeable mood swings or SAD (Seasonal Affective Disorder), enjoy a second cup of warm cinnamon tea near mid afternoon.

Moderation and common sense have always been the key to successful living. Scientists tell us that, for optimum health, we need tiny amounts of hundreds of compounds, many of which have not yet been identified. Exactly how the body uses some of these trace elements remains a medical mystery. We do know that if there is an imbalance of vitamins or minerals the body will react to the shortage. For a serious illness, or little problems that do not go away, you need a physician. For the aches and pains that make up everyday living, let old-time remedies help you along your way.

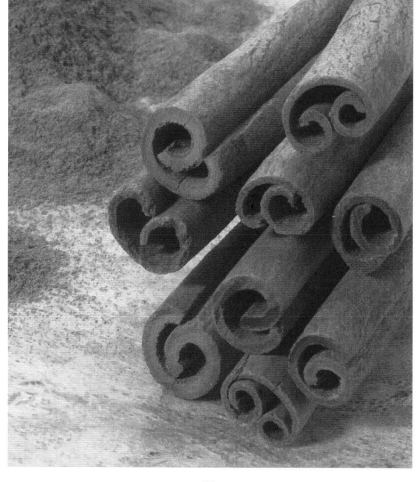

CHAPTER SIX

On the Horizon:
Cinnamon's Future
In the Medical World

While much is known about cinnamon's amazing use as a medicinal spice, much has yet to be discovered. In many ways, scientists have only scratched the surface in incorporating cinnamon into the medical world. Countless studies are ongoing endeavoring to learn more about the "how's" and "why's" in regard to cinnamon's effectiveness when used to battle a host of the body's conditions and ailments.

Scientists hold great hope that cinnamon will one day be proven to help treat some of the most baffling conditions the human body can face. Some of this research includes looking into cinnamon's effect on:

- Alzheimer patients
- Dementia
- Multiple sclerosis
- Ulcers
- Obesity

What do we know at this point?

The science of cinnamon as a medicinal aid is still in its infancy as far as conclusions go. But studies are ongoing all around the world with several of these studies beginning to show great promise.

A study conducted by the U.S. Department of Agriculture has concluded that cinnamon extract can work to help reduce many of the risk factors that accompany those suffering from heart disease and diabetes. In this particular study, 22 patients considered to be pre-diabetics took part in a 12 week clinical trial using cinnamon. Eleven of the patients were given 250 mg of cinnamon extract twice a day over the 12 week period, while the other 11 participants were given a placebo.

Fasting blood tests were conducted at the beginning of the experiment, and also the halfway point and at once again at the conclusion of the test. At the conclusion of the experiment, both sets of patients had blood sugar levels tested. The results of these tests indicated an improvement of between 13% and 23% of the antioxidant levels in the body. This was attributed to a drop in glucose levels.

Based on this evidence, additional studies will need to be conducted to learn how this drop in glucose levels can be safely used to combat both obesity and diabetes.

In another study, this from Rush University Medical Center, found that the metabolism-altering effects of cinnamon, sodium benzoate, can actually work to block the body's chemicals that promote inflammation within the body. Even more interesting is the ability to activate the body's glial cells which are known to destroy myelin sheath in multiple sclerosis sufferers.

It is thought that cinnamon's anti-inflammatory properties may work to lessen or stop glial cell production within the body that cause the destruction of brain cells in patients with multiple sclerosis.

The *Journal of Immunology* published a study in which various doses of sodium benzoate were added to the drinking water of animals. Over time, the study showed a 70% reduction in multiple sclerosis scores in the tested animals. Researchers are studying ways that eventually may incorporate cinnamon as a treatment for those suffering from this debilitating disease.

Beth Israel Deaconess Medical Center recently published an article featuring the exciting test results of cinnamon's effectiveness on an array of conditions. Cinnamon hosts several unique properties, such as being antibacterial, antifungal and antiparasitic, which is believed to make it a potent remedy against common head lice, thrust and even yeast infections. Animal studies have indicated that cinnamon may offer potential benefits to those suffering from diabetes. And conclusions from two different animals research projects indicate that cinnamon extract, when taken orally, may work to prevent stomach ulcers.

While this is certainly exciting news for the medical world, additional studies still need to corroborate the research, and studies need to move from animal based testing to human trials. But so far, the results are moving in the right direction.

In other research, more than eight studies on human participants established the effectiveness of cassia cinnamon in stabilizing insulin levels. In these tests, cassia cinnamon showed a therapeutic effect on the reduction of fasting blood glucose levels in participants by more than 10%. An additional study indicated that cinnamon reduced total cholesterol levels, LDL ("bad") cholesterol and triglycerides.

Numerous studies into cinnamon's effect on weight loss have been conducted world wide. Research seems to indicate that as little as a teaspoon of cinnamon per day can positively effect the body's metabolism, making weight loss easier. Cinnamon creates a chemical reaction within the body that works to increase the body's metabolic rate, which in turn causes the body to burn fat faster. Several foods and spices are known for speeding up metabolism, but cinnamon and cayenne pepper are significantly more potent than others for this purpose.

When cinnamon has been consumed, it combines with natural occurring chemicals within the body to cause a thermogenic reaction. It is this chemical reaction that hastens the body's natural metabolic rate and speeds up weight loss.

Cinnamon also maintains healthy fasting blood sugar levels. This is an important aspect of weight loss, as spiking blood sugar levels can induce food cravings. These cravings often wind up as unwanted calories.

Another aspect of cinnamon as it relates to weight loss is its ability to control plaque and fat deposits in the arteries. Studies have shown that arterial fat deposits and plaque can also make weight loss more difficult in patients who are obese.

Pharmacological studies are also being conducted on cinnamon's effectiveness at addressing other conditions such as helicobacter pylori infections, stimulation of the olfactory cortex of the brain, and even oral fungal infections in HIV patients and others with compromised immune systems.

Tel Aviv University in Israel has conducted numerous studies on laboratory mice and learned that a specific chemical found occurring naturally in cinnamon worked not only to prevent the development of Alzheimer's disease, but may also work to cure the disease in those already suffering from it. Also discovered was the potential for cinnamon to inhibit the activity of what is known as "coated" viruses, such as influenza and herpes.

Professor Michael Ovadia headed the research team from Tel Aviv University, and the University went on to issue a patent on the cinnamon composition it discovered along with its use as a dietary supplement.

He states, "The discovery is very exciting because, while there are companies that develop synthetic compounds that inhibit Alzheimer's, the discovered substance is not a drug with side effects, but rather a safe and natural substance that people consume for generations."

MD Anderson Cancer Center has also conducted research into cinnamon's ability fight cancer cells. Studies in mice reported that cinnamon nutraceuticals, the part of cinnamon that actually provides health benefits, inhibited the inflammation of cancer cell pathways. This discovery is crucially important in cancer research as scientists now know that inflammation is directly linked to the formation and spread of cancer.

The Gwangju Institute of Science and Technology in the Korea conducted a 2010 study on the anti-tumor effects of cinnamon. Cinnamon extract was not only shown to inhibit the growth of cancer cells, but also the spread of cancer. This study was conducive to several types of cancer including melanoma, lymphoma, colorectal cancer and cervical cancer.

Professor Bharat Aggarwal from the Department of Therapeutics at MD Anderson states that, "The medicinal value of spices, such as cinnamon, has been recognized for centuries by a variety of cultures," Aggarwal says. "Even so, much of their potential has only been realized over the past 50 years. We are just scratching the surface of how spices can impact cancer. The research being done is promising."

Aggarwal also believes the incorporation of cinnamon into the diet is a good thing, with many potential health benefits.

This research is by no means complete, and will take many more years of study to come to a definitive conclusion. And in many of these results, science still needs to make the jump between animal studies and human trials. But preliminary results are exciting and lead one to believe that cinnamon may have more potent effects on the human body than anyone ever thought possible. Continuing research is certainly warranted and one should stay alert as science looks at ways to incorporate positive test results into making treatments using cinnamon readily available to the awaiting public.

For those suffering from the effects of these devastating diseases, do not lose hope! Help may be on the horizon.

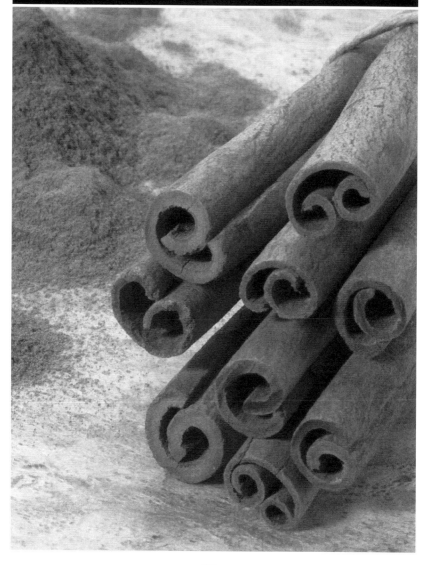

CHAPTER SEVEN
Health and Beauty

Throughout the ages, cinnamon was a treasured spice and commodity. It was greatly sought after as a valuable spice for flavoring dishes, but also for its many medicinal properties and preservations qualities. But as time went on, cinnamon was discovered to have uses as a wonder-filled beauty agent.

It may come as a surprise that cinnamon is not just used for cooking or natural home health remedies. Cinnamon is also a wonderful, widely untapped natural beauty enhancer.

Did you know cinnamon is a common ingredient in some of today's best known manufactured cosmetics? Cinnamon has been found in a wide variety of products, including:

- Lipstick
- Rouges
- Bath salts and oils
- Hair lighteners
- Bronzers

Cinnamon's uses in the cosmetic industry are amazing. The very properties that make cinnamon an excellent agent for home remedies, also make it a fantastic beauty agent. Cinnamon contains unique properties such as being an:

- Antioxidant
- Antibacterial
- Antimicrobial
- Antiseptic
- Analgesic

- Astringent
- Aphrodisiac

Cinnamon also has some of the most widely used aromatic and therapeutic fragrances around. Cinnamon oils are used extensively in aromatherapy sessions and holistic treatment approaches. It can be used to calms the senses and alleviate tension.

New research studies show that cinnamon vapors can even enhance memory and thought patterns. Studies were done on participants with specific memory tasks. The participants were asked to complete a series of memory tasks. Some of these tasks were done under the influence of cinnamon aroma. Other tasks were not. Those tasks that were done with a cinnamon fragrance had better memory results than those that did not. This is just another reason why, in addition to its calming qualities, cinnamon makes a fantastic aromatherapy agent.

Cinnamon can also be found in a wide array of beauty products, with new items constantly being added to the market. A few of these beauty products include:

- Bath gels
- Lotions
- Hair care products and rinses
- Massage oils
- Toothpastes
- Gum
- Candies
- Cleansing agents

- Breath fresheners
- Mouthwashes
- Perfumes
- Body sprays

The natural richness of cinnamon's coloring is the obvious choice of additions in many rouges and blush cosmetics. It adds a natural touch of color, and also brings antiseptic and antimicrobial aspects to make up.

Cinnamon is used not only as a colorant, but more surprisingly as a plumping agent in some of the best lipsticks and glosses available. The potency of cinnamon as an ingredient placed on delicate lips can cause a light tingling feeling. This "tingling" is actually a very mild, though not harmful, irritant that causes sensitive lip tissues to lightly swell. The swelling mechanism is sold as lip plumping action in many of today's lip enhancers.

With cinnamon being so widely used in the beauty industry, why not use those very same discoveries in our own daily home beauty regimens? And, cinnamon has countless benefits over its commercially manufactured beauty counterpart. Cinnamon is:

- Inexpensive
- Readily available
- Non-toxic
- Chemical-free
- Not tested on animals
- Environmentally friendly
- All natural

Words of caution

Just a few brief words of caution when using cinnamon as a natural beauty enhancer.

Cinnamon is a great additive for coloring hair or using as a blush or bronzing agent. But the very quality that makes it so wonderful, also deserves a moment of pause. Remember that cinnamon can temporarily stain shirt colors or bathroom towels as you are applying or mixing your beauty products. Care should be taken to avoid contact with anything you do not wish to look or smell like cinnamon!

Also, cinnamon can be irritating to some people with sensitive skin. Be sure and test your home made beauty product before using it on vast amounts of skin.

In addition, cinnamon oil, while wonderfully potent for its aroma and as a therapeutic massage oil, is cinnamon in its most concentrated form. You may wish to dilute the oil in warm water or another liquid substance to prevent irritating delicate skin tissue.

Ready, set, go!

Enough talk. Time to begin discovering the amazing wonders cinnamon has to offer your skin, hair and anywhere else you would like to experience its unique effects.

Give a few of these ideas a try, and then step out and be adventurous! Discover your own ways cinnamon can enhance your natural beauty!

Cinnamon hair lightener

Place a quarter cup of your favorite conditioner in a small bowl. Add a couple of tablespoons of honey along with three or four tablespoons of cinnamon. Mix together until thoroughly combined. Wash your hair like normal and towel dry. Do not dry completely. Add mixture to hair a few sections at a time. Be sure to apply all the way to the roots. Wrap hair in plastic wrap or a towel and rest under a warm dryer or heat for about thirty minutes. Rinse conditioner out with warm water to reveal highlighted hair.

Hair streaking or tinting

To achieve those beautiful summer streaks in your hair. Try this cinnamon concoction:

Combine one or two tablespoons of honey with four tablespoons of cinnamon. With a comb or pick, gently lift pieces of hair desiring tint. Brush the honey and cinnamon mixture onto well placed hair strands and allow to sit in the sun or beneath a warm dryer for 20 or 30 minutes. Rinse mixture out of hair. The combination of cinnamon along with the natural lightening effects of honey will result in light, but beautiful summer streaking.

Cleansing wash

For skin clear of acne or other unwanted blemishes, try this formula. Steep a cinnamon stick in a cup of hot water for ten minutes. After the water has cooled to a safe, warm temperature, use it to cleanse your face and open blocked pores.

Acne

Use this concoction to treat stubborn acne.

1/4 cup honey
1 tsp cinnamon

Blend the honey and cinnamon together. Dab a bit on stubborn acne before going to bed each night. Rinse well with warm water in the morning, and in a few weeks the skin will be clear of unsightly pimples.

This remedy is very gentle and can be used as often as you like without the need to worry about irritating sensitive facial skin tissue.

Blackheads

To make a homemade, natural blackhead remover, try this:

Combine equal parts ground cinnamon and lime juice, mixing into a paste. Apply paste to face and allow to dry. Gently rinse cinnamon solution from face to cleanse and remove blackheads.

Soft skin

1/4 cup honey
1 tbsp cinnamon
2 cups water

Mix well and drink a quarter cup of this mixture several times a day. Your skin will stay soft and youthful looking.

Bronzing powder

Make your own bronzing powder, unique to your very own skin color, with a wonderful combination of cinnamon and nutmeg. Combine one tablespoon of cornstarch, two teaspoons cinnamon and a half teaspoon cocoa. Put all the ingredients into a small jar and mix together. Use a cotton ball, sponge or cosmetic puff to apply on the skin.

For darker shades of color, add a touch more cinnamon or cocoa to the cornstarch.

Blusher

Try making a simple blushing powder by mixing one tablespoon of cornstarch with two teaspoons of cinnamon. Mix together and apply to cheek bones with a cosmetic brush.

Adjust the intensity of the cinnamon blusher by adding or subtracting the amount of cinnamon mixed with cornstarch to your own personal preference.

Contour powder

For a bolder contour powder, try this mixture. In a small container blend together equal parts cornstarch and cinnamon. Use a cosmetic or contour brush to apply to hollow area beneath cheekbones.

As before, don't forget you can change the intensity of the contour powder by adjusting the ratio of cornstarch to cinnamon.

Have slightly darker skin tones? Add a pinch of cocoa powder to darken the effect.

Massage oil

Add a few drops of cinnamon extract or oil to your favorite massage oil for a calming, aromatic effect. In some countries, the aroma of cinnamon is also considered an aphrodisiac.

Take a clean washcloth and dip into a bowl of warm water in which a few drops of cinnamon oil has been placed. Wring out your cloth and use to bring light refreshment to your skin.

Plump lips

Want fuller lips but aren't interested in cosmetic surgery or injections? Cinnamon's might be your answer.

Many cosmetic manufacturers use cinnamon in their lip products to enhance lip appearance. It seems the cinnamaldehyde found naturally in cinnamon causes delicate lip tissue to enlarge and swell slightly.

Apply a cinnamon-added lip gloss to your lips for fuller, more plump lips. Expect to feel a slight tingling feeling, as this is the cinnamaldehyde at work.

Cinnamon bath

Add a few drops of cinnamon oil to your evening bath for a wonderful aromatic sensation. This will go a long way to help put an end to tensions and enhance sleep. It is also great for calming the senses and aiding in relaxation.

If cinnamon oil is unavailable, cinnamon extract works as a great substitution for baths. Just be sure to add more extract than you would use oil, as the extract is more diluted than cinnamon oil.

Insect repellent

DEET, or its full chemical name N,N-Diethyl-meta-toluamide is the active ingredient in most store purchased insect repellents. DEET is a strong chemical which was originally used by the Army in World War II. Cautions have demanded that DEET be avoided in direct contact with the skin, or on clothing where it might remain near delicate skin tissue.

So, do we have an alternative? Cinnamon, of course!

Want to try a more natural approach to repelling insects? Try adding a few drops of cinnamon oil to your favorite lotion and apply directly to your skin before heading outdoors. Unscented lotions seem to work better, as scented lotions can be attractive to nasty bugs and insects.

Kill mosquito larvae instantly by combining a small amount of cinnamon oil with an equal amount of catnip oil. This combination is not only deadly to the larvae, but is environmentally friendly and safe for both children and pets.

Make your own insect spray. Add a few drops of cinnamon oil to a small spray bottle full of water. Before heading outside, give your clothing a quick spray of this mixture to keep mosquitoes away.

Cinnamon oil may also be applied to the skin after it has been diluted with water or another diluting agent. While cinnamon oil is extremely effective in combating insects in its purest form, its concentrated form can be irritating on sensitive skin tissue if used straight out of the bottle.

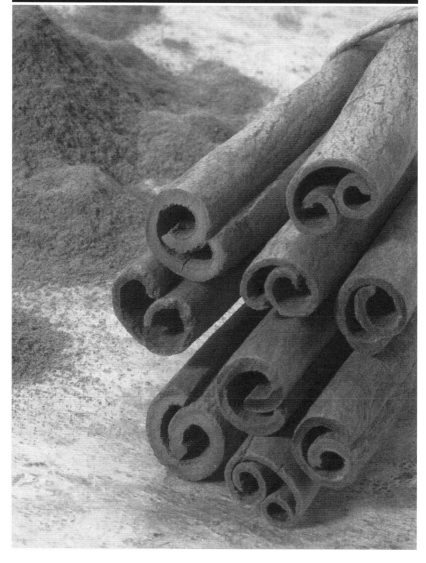

CHAPTER EIGHT
Around the Home

Who doesn't love the fresh, spiced scent and aroma of natural cinnamon! And with all cinnamon's amazing properties, it makes the perfect addition for around-the-home use! Not only can cinnamon tackle some of your more interesting issues around the home, but also leaves behind a fresh, clean smell to brighten any home.

You'll find many uses for trading in your old, store bought chemically-based products and replacing them will all natural cinnamon.

Consumers are also becoming more savvy and shying away from harsh chemicals. For instance, why purchase a chemically formulated air freshener which only masks household odors? Cinnamon not only leaves a home smelling fresh and clean, but also contains natural anti bacterial agents which can be used to combat the source of the odor – not just cover it up!

And, as time goes on we are becoming more aware of the environmental impact commercially produced household products have. Consider this:

- The manufacturing of not only the chemical-based products, but also the plastic bottles themselves, creates toxic pollutions added to our environment.

- Each year, millions of these plastic bottles and containers wind up in landfills.

- Many of these chemicals have been proven to harm wildlife and their surrounding environments as they are added to our waste system.

- Chemical run off wastes emitted from discarded cleaning bottles trickled their way into our streams and wetlands which, in turn, affect the fish and game population.

- Household freshener and cleaning products can leave behind unwanted chemical residue in our living and eating areas.

Another aspect of turning to a more natural approach around the home is cost consideration. Each of these home uses can be made yourself, saving countless dollars on the family budget! You can even try purchasing cinnamon in larger bulk quantities for even greater savings on the pocketbook!

Keep in mind that because in the case of using cinnamon around the home, or even out in the garden on plants and other vegetation, we are not looking to reap the same health benefits we may be looking for in our natural home health remedies. Any cinnamon will do for these applications. You do not need to purchase the more expensive Ceylon cinnamon. In fact, even "old" cinnamon that has been found buried in an old drawer or spice rack will do just fine! It's a great way to put older, forgotten bottles of cinnamon to great use instead of throwing them out.

Cinnamon outdoors
So many times its easy to reach for a chemical bug spray or repellent. But when we are dealing with garden plants that may ultimately wind up on our dinner tables, it

is best to steer clear of any harmful chemicals which might compromise the health of the plant or its vegetation. Who would want to eat a tomato from plants sprayed or treated with dangerous chemicals? In these cases, it is always best to go natural!

Cinnamon can be the perfect solution to this delicate balance.

Cinnamon has been found to be a harsh irritant for bugs and insects. They don't seem to like its potency and are easily repelled by it. However, plant life is equally unaffected by the spice. This makes cinnamon a unique and surprising choice for home gardening problems.

And obviously, cinnamon is fully natural, contains a healthful mixture of vitamins, minerals and essential nutrients, and lacks all of the dangerous side effects which may come with the use of store bought gardening chemicals and treatment products.

Instead, try a few of these gardening solutions the next time you are tempted to reach for a store bought chemical product:

Plant fungus treatment
Cinnamon's anti-fungal properties work wonders on both preventing and treating plants for fungus.

Treat a favorite indoor or outdoor gardening plant with this cinnamon remedy to rid it of nagging fungus. Take a spray bottle filled with water and gently damped the affected leaves. Next, sprinkle a little cinnamon directly onto the leaves and allow to dry for 7 to 10 days. After that time, leaves should be cleared up and free from fungus.

Try to prevent fungus from occurring at all when starting new plants. After seeds have been planted, or new starts have been put in the ground, sprinkle a little cinnamon on the top of the potting soil to prevent fungus from starting at all.

Be sure and dust new plant shoots with a light sprinkling of cinnamon as soon as they spring up from the ground. This will both prevent fungus from developing, and keep insects from attacking the delicate young plants.

Aphids and other plant destroying insects

Keep ravaging aphids and other plant eating insects at bay by sprinkling cinnamon around the base of the plants. It's okay if some of the cinnamon gets sprinkled on a few leaves as well.

Make your own insect repelling liquid spray by combining a cup of water with a few teaspoons of ground cinnamon. Use this to spray on and around plants to protect them from harmful, leaf-eating insects.

Want to try something a little more out-of-the-box? Try planting a few cinnamon basil plants in between precious garden plants like tomatoes or peppers to keep insects away altogether. While cinnamon basil is not true cinnamon, it does contain some of the same properties that give cinnamon its aroma and potency, and can often times mimic the benefits of real cinnamon. This can be an effective way of keeping insects away, and also providing an extra herb in your garden at the same time!

Have a favorite tree or bush in your outdoor landscape that is being over ridden with bugs and insects? Try working a cinnamon tree somewhere in the landscape. The cinnamon tree will remain free of critters while the surrounding plants will remain unaffected as well.

So next time you reach for that air freshener or store bought household cleaning product, try one of these natural solutions first!

Air freshener

Love cinnamon's amazing aroma, and want more of it around your home? Why not try making your own natural air freshener, free of harmful chemicals and completely environmentally safe.

Take a plastic spray bottle and fill it full of tap water. Add a few drops of cinnamon oil or cinnamon extract and shake it all together. Use the spray around the home to give rooms a clean, refreshing aroma.

Place a little ground cinnamon into your vacuum cleaner bag to give off a wonderful cinnamon fragrance with every use.

For another simple air freshener, heat a small bowl of water in the microwave. When finished, add a few drops of cinnamon oil or extract to the warm water and place bowl on a table or counter top.

To make your own hanging air freshener for a closet, car or other small space, try making your own hanging air freshener. Take a piece of heavy felt or thick card stock.

Feel free to make a friendly shape out of the felt or stock and punch a hole in the top. Use a length of yarn or string to tie to the card and make it into a hanging loop. Now place a few drops of either cinnamon oil or extract directly onto the card and hang to freshen a car or closet.

Feeling more adventurous? Make a longer lasting hanging air freshener. In a small bowl, combine one half cup cinnamon, one half cup applesauce, one teaspoon salt, one tablespoon cornstarch and two heaping tablespoons of white or craft glue. Using your hands, combine all ingredients until you have achieved a soft, moldable dough. Roll out into 1/4" thickness and use your favorite cookie cutters to cut the dough into shapes. Using a pencil or straw, poke a hole near the top of each shape, allowing the hole to go all the way thru the shape. Place on a piece of parchment paper and allow the shaped dough to remain undisturbed for several days until completely dry. String a piece of yarn or ribbon through each hole and tie into a bow or knot and use to hang around your home.

Cinnamon potpourri
Make your own amazing cinnamon potpourri using a few of these amazing recipes.

Combine four cinnamon sticks, broken into pieces, with one quarter cup whole allspice, several torn bay leaves, one quarter cup lemon or orange peels and a few drops of cinnamon oil. Mix together and store in a tightly covered jar for two weeks to blend the aromas together. Then simply remove the lid and enjoy around the home.

For another wonderful potpourri, try this dry mixture. Pick a cup or two of flowers from around your home. Roses, Queen Anne's lace and hydrangeas all work well. Any flower that will dry well and leave you with a beautifully colored dried flower can be used. Place flower heads on a paper towel and allow to dry for a couple of weeks. When flowers are completely dry, place them in a decorative glass container and add several cinnamon sticks, broken into small pieces, along with a handful of whole cloves and a few drops of cinnamon oil. Make sure to stir it together and place lid on jar. Allow aromas to meld together for a few days. When ready, just remove the lid and place your new decorative jar of cinnamon potpourri around your home.

Ready for that beautiful Christmas aroma for the holidays? Try putting a cup or two of apple cider on the stove along with a handful of cloves and a couple of cinnamon sticks. Allow this mixture to simmer during your holiday celebrations to spread a wonderful aroma throughout your home.

These potpourri ideas are just the beginning! Don't be afraid to try your own aromatic combinations. Each potpourri concoction can be as unique as the person you are. Along with your dried flowers and cinnamon sticks and oils, feel free to explore other essential oils and extracts in combination with cinnamon to arrive at your own, personalized fragrance. A few additions that might work well with cinnamon include lemon, orange, lavender and even vanilla. The combinations are endless! Try a few of your own favorites for a special scent.

Natural food preserver

Once, cinnamon was used as a preservative for foods. Today, we know that we can add a stick of cinnamon to flour or cornmeal to deter insect activity.

Also consider adding cinnamon to flavored dishes as a way to preserve dishes that may not be served immediately.

Cinnamon dye to fabric

Cinnamon can be used to dye fabrics in an amazing array of shades, colors and uses. Try these dye and staining concoctions and then use them as a springboard to discover your own colors and uses. You'll find that cinnamon can be used in many ways to bring color to bland fabric.

Before getting started, here are a few tips to keep in mind whenever using cinnamon or other spices and herbs as a fabric dye:

- The longer a fabric stays immersed in the solution, the darker and more intense the color will become.

- For smooth, even color saturation, soak fabrics in clean water prior to dying.

- For a more mottled or splotchy effect, place dry fabrics directly into the dying solution without the clean water wetting first.

- Fabric can be hung up to dry for a more even look, or wadded up and wrapped in rubber bands for a more mottled or tie dyed effect.

- While dyed fabric is still wet, try sprinkling with cinnamon and allowing to completely dry. After drying, cinnamon can be brushed off, or lightly washed off. This will give the fabric dark red spots intermingled with the colored fabric for a unique look.

- Consider blending additional spices for a multi-colored look to your fabrics. Boil several pots of water, each with a different spice or herb, and dip different portions of the fabric into the colored water. Ideal spices to try include cinnamon, mustard, ginger, paprika and thyme.

- Also try using a combination of colorful mashed berries or spinach leaves for additional color options.

To give new fabrics that antiqued, aged look, try this mixture. Combine five cups of water with one or two cups of instant coffee grounds. Bring mixture to a boil over medium heat. Remove mixture from stove and add one or two teaspoons of ground cinnamon. Mix thoroughly. Place a yard or so of fabric into the solution and allow to sit until the cloth reaches the desired color or hue. Hang the fabric to dry in a safe place, keeping in mind that any drips from the wet fabric might stain the area it comes in contact with.

One additional note: the fabric will lighten as it dries, so stay aware of that as you are deciding when to remove the fabric from the color bath. Fabric color should be checked after 15 or 20 minutes, but can be kept immersed in the liquid for more than an hour until it reaches it full intensity.

Ready for another way to die fabric with cinnamon? Fill a small pot with water and add a quarter cup of cinnamon. Bring to a boil and remove from heat. Place fabric into the pot and allow to sit until desired color and intensity is reached.

Moth repellent

Replace mothballs in your closet with this homemade recipe. Combine equal parts broken cinnamon sticks and peppercorns and place into small bags or sachets. Place around closet.

Cinnamon diffuser

Drop a little cinnamon oil on a cool light bulb and allow to dry. Turn the light on. As the bulb's heat begins to warm the oil, your room will be filled with a wonderful cinnamon fragrance.

Place a few drops of cinnamon oil on candles, heating radiator or heating vents and allow the heating process to unleash the oil's fresh aroma.

Fresh, fragrant decorations

Tie a few fresh cinnamon sticks together using a beautiful ribbon or bow and hang it near the front door of your home. Entering guests will be treated to the fresh, fragrant aroma of luscious cinnamon upon coming through the threshold.

Place several whole cinnamon sticks in a shallow glass dish or decorative decanter along with a handful of cranberries. Place decanter in the center of a table to enjoy.

Make your own beautiful, fragrant holiday centerpiece that will be the envy of all your friends. Begin with a small pillar candle, several inches in width and height. Take cinnamon sticks and place all the way around the candle, completely encasing the outside of the candle. Using a piece of twine or pretty ribbon, tie the cinnamon sticks to the candle. Place on a tray and surround with cranberries, or even several other cinnamon surrounded candles for a gorgeous centerpiece.

Tie cinnamon sticks to satin flowers and plants throughout the house.

Hide a cinnamon stick or two above doorway frames and arches around your home for the holidays. Guests will be reminded of Christmas everywhere they go.

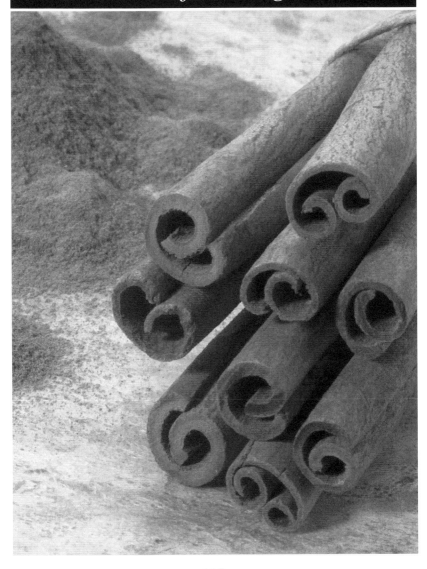

CHAPTER NINE
Cinnamon for Weight Loss

We all know cinnamon is a fantastically delicious spice used in many of the most coveted recipes from all over the world. And, we have discovered countless uses for cinnamon as a natural home health remedy shown successful in combating everything from an open cut to lowering cholesterol and stabilizing insulin levels in diabetes patients. But did you know researchers have also found cinnamon useful in promoting weight loss?

How cinnamon works in weight loss

Cinnamon is able to achieve weight loss through several specific chemical functions.

- **Metabolism** Cinnamon's many medicinal properties work to stabilize metabolism and hasten weight loss. Cinnamon has been found to create a chemical reaction with the body that works to increase metabolism causing the body to burn fat faster. While many foods are renown for speeding up metabolism, cinnamon and cayenne pepper are significantly more potent than others for this purpose.

  When cinnamon has been consumed, it combines with natural occurring chemicals within the body to cause a thermogenic reaction. It is this chemical reaction that hastens the body's natural metabolic rate and speeds up weight loss.

- **Stabilizing blood sugar levels thru insulin** Keeping blood sugar levels is imperative for weight loss. When blood sugar levels rise and fall dependant on meals or snacks eaten throughout the day, weight loss becomes very difficult.

A study conducted by the prestigious Mayo Clinic found that blood sugar levels in patients suffering from type-2 diabetes can be helped regulated with cinnamon. These studies concluded that eating cinnamon two times a day over the period of several months increased the body's insulin levels, therefore stabilizing blood sugar levels.

When the body's blood sugar is stabilized, the body experiences less hunger cravings. And, obviously, less hunger cravings throughout the day results in less calories and greater loss of excess weight.

- **Cholesterol** Research through the American Diabetes Association has shown that cinnamon works to reduce total cholesterol levels, dangerous triglycerides and LDL (low density lipoprotein) or "bad" cholesterol. It is thought that fat and cholesterol built up in the arteries can hamper weight loss. By working to reduce cholesterol levels and fat and cholesterol build up in the blood stream, the body is free to burn fat and calories as it should...even stubborn belly fat.

The Cinnamon Diet

You may have heard of the latest trend among dieters, called the Cinnamon Diet. Maybe you've seen it on the cover of a magazine or heard it discussed among television doctors. It has even appeared in *Woman's World* magazine.

It has been referred to as the "belly fat pill" touting dramatic inches of stubborn belly fat lost after consuming cinnamon in the diet. Claims have been made that this simple diet can help you drop nearly 10 pounds in a single week!

So what is the Cinnamon Diet? Is there any truth behind the hype? Is it possible this diet can live up to all its supposed to?

Experts tell us that cinnamon can lower blood sugar levels by almost 30%. Lower blood sugar levels can help speed up the body's metabolism and induce weight loss. The theory behind the Cinnamon Diet is to speed up the body's metabolic rate, cut dangerous cholesterol, LDL and triglyceride numbers and stabilize glucose levels. All of this, say the experts, works to make you lose more weight, at a faster rate. (On a side note, these are also identical reasons diabetics ingest cinnamon to help manage diabetes.)

The Cinnamon Diet is based on the premise of ingesting one teaspoon of cinnamon, spread throughout the day. For some, this translates into 1/4 teaspoon in the morning for breakfast, a half teaspoon with your lunchtime meal, and the final quarter teaspoon with dinner. Cinnamon can come in any form, and does not need to be sprinkled over food, or mixed into tea, although these are both fine choices. You may also include baked goods which contain cinnamon, or dishes, such as cinnamon rice, where cinnamon plays a part.

These latter ideas are excellent ways to incorporate cinnamon into your diet plan, but can be a little tricky when trying to track the actual amount of cinnamon consumed.

Some diet users either mix a quarter teaspoon of cinnamon into their drink, or combine the cinnamon with a teaspoon or so of honey and eat it. Any of these suggestions will work well for this particular diet.

Many users of the Cinnamon Diet begin noticing results after just five days, with weight loss ranging anywhere from 2 to 10 pounds the first week! Obviously, not everyone will experience the same benefits of the Cinnamon Diet, but it may be worth exploring!

So far, the Cinnamon Diet appears to be living up to its promise of noticeable weight loss results. Let's watch as more information becomes available on this one!

Which type of cinnamon works best?

So, which type of cinnamon works best for weight loss? The jury is still out on a definitive answer to whether Ceylon or cassia cinnamon works best. Many natural health experts claim that Ceylon cinnamon is the most effective route for faster weight loss, but others disagree.

For those people interested in weight loss who are also monitoring coumadin levels due to other health conditions, Ceylon could be the wisest choice. Ceylon cinnamon, as discussed in previous chapters, does seem to possess the most health benefits, although in some cases the differences may not be as noticeable as people once thought.

Regardless of which type of cinnamon you decide to use, the key to using cinnamon for weight loss is steady use over the period of 8 to 12 weeks.

How much cinnamon makes a difference

Studies show that as little as one and a half teaspoons a day can make a marked improvement in increased metabolism and overall weight loss. This amount of cinnamon can be ingested in any number of ways. Enjoying a series of edibles in which cinnamon is an ingredient throughout the day is thought to have the same amazing outcome of consuming the cinnamon in one sitting, drinking a warm cup of tea in which the entire one and a half teaspoons has been added.

And the results appear to be identical whether the cinnamon is baked, soaked or steeped, or sprinkled fresh over your favorite food. Cooking and baking apparently does not reduce the effectiveness of cinnamon's weight loss abilities.

One thought about using cinnamon in baked goods to reach the target amount of one and a half teaspoons. If weight loss is your goal, consuming cinnamon in baked goods such as cinnamon buns and cookies could be counterproductive. While cinnamon's effectiveness in being cooked is not compromised, the extra calories derived from baked goods makes weight loss difficult. Look for more appropriate ways of incorporating cinnamon in which you are not adding unwanted additional calories to your daily totals.

A few of these suggestions might include:

- Cinnamon over a half cup of applesauce

- Enjoy a warm cup of your favorite tea, enhanced with cinnamon

- While it might be difficult to monitor the amount of actual cinnamon consumed, try swirling a cinnamon stick in your favorite diet cola

- Try an afternoon snack of sliced apples sprinkled with cinnamon

- A little yogurt sprinkled with cinnamon can be an enjoyable, nutritious treat

- Start your day off right with a little cinnamon mixed in with honey and spread on a bagel or slice of toast

- Cinnamon and cottage cheese or oatmeal make a delicious combination

Try a few of these recipes for adding cinnamon to your daily health regimen for better weight loss.

Spreads and Dips

Cinnamon Honey Spread

Try this simple but tasty spread as a no-hassle way of increasing your cinnamon intake.

1 tbsp honey
1 tsp cinnamon

Combine both ingredients and spread over a bagel or slice of toast.

Fall Cinnamon Spread

Here is a special cinnamon spread that can be made in a small batch ahead of time, and used as desired throughout the week.

1/2 cup butter or low calorie spread, softened
3 tbsp brown sugar
1 tsp cinnamon
Pinch of nutmeg

Beat butter or spread substitute until creamy and add remaining ingredients. Mix all ingredients together in a small bowl until thoroughly combined. Cover and place in refrigerator and use throughout the week as often as you like.

Low Fat Cinnamon Dip

Make a batch of this cinnamon dip to enjoy with various fresh fruits. Apples, grapes, pineapple, strawberries, kiwi and watermelon are excellent choices to accompany this dip.

1/2 cup low fat vanilla yogurt
3 tbsp applesauce
1/2 tsp cinnamon
1/4 tsp nutmeg

Blend all ingredients together and serve cold with fresh fruit.

Healthy Snacks

Cinnamon Granola

This is an amazing granola packed with nutrients you can enjoy any time of day.

4 cup quick oats
2 cup water
3/4 cup brown sugar
2 tbsp cinnamon
Pinch of ground cloves

Combine oats, brown sugar, cinnamon and cloves in a bowl, thoroughly coating oats. Add water and mix thoroughly. Spread mixture out on a baking sheet in an even layer. Bake at 325° for 20-30 minutes until dried out and crunchy.

Low Fat Cinnamon Chips

Looking for a tasty, fun chip to snack on while watching your favorite movie?

5 flour tortillas
1 tbsp sugar
1/2 tbsp cinnamon
Cooking spray

Combine sugar and cinnamon in a small bowl. Place tortillas on a baking sheet and lightly coat with cooking spray. Using a pizza cutter, cut tortillas into wedges and sprinkle with cinnamon mixture. Bake at 400° for 8 to 10 minutes, or until lightly crispy.

Healthful Nuts and Spice

This is a fantastic recipe and excellent for not only bringing additional cinnamon into your diet, but also a variety of nutritious fruits and nuts.

2 cups of your favorite nuts (almonds, peanuts, etc.)
1 cups dried fruit (raisins, dried cranberries, etc.)
1/3 cup honey
1 tsp cinnamon
pinch of cloves
Coconut flakes, if desired

In a bowl, combine all ingredients, gently stirring until nuts and fruit are thoroughly coated in honey and cinnamon. Spread coated nuts on a baking sheet and bake for 20 minutes at 375°. Enjoy!

Low Fat Cinnamon Toast

Here is a wonderful alternative to regular cinnamon toast.

Slice of bread
Low fat butter flavored cooking spray
1 tbsp sugar
1 tsp cinnamon

Combine sugar and cinnamon, and set aside. Spray slice of bread with cooking spray and toast in a frying pan over medium heat until toasted, being sure to flip toast and cook on both sides. When finished, sprinkle with sugar cinnamon mixture and enjoy.

Low Fat Cinnamon Raisin English Muffins

This is a wonderful recipe for a low fat version of the English muffin, cinnamon-style.

1/3 cup warm water (about 110°)
1 tbsp sugar
1 packet dry yeast
1 cup skim (fat free) milk
2 cup flour
1/2 tsp salt
2 tsp cinnamon
1/2 cup raisins
Cooking spray

Pour warm water into a bowl. Add sugar, stirring to dissolve completely. Sprinkle yeast over top of sugar water and set aside, undisturbed. Do not stir. Allow yeast mixture to rest for 10 minutes until it blooms (foams).

While yeast is blooming, combine flour, salt, cinnamon and skim milk. Add yeast mixture and stir until smooth and ingredients are completely incorporated. Gently stir in raisins. Cover dough with plastic wrap and let rise on the counter for one hour.

Coat a griddle with cooking spray and heat to medium high. One quarter cup at a time, drop dough by spoonfuls onto griddle and cook until muffins are very slightly browned. Turn over and repeat on the other side. Muffins will appear slightly dry.

For even more cinnamon enjoyment, serve with cinnamon honey spread.

Drinks

Cinnamon Tea

Delicious, warm cinnamon tea is a delightful way to enjoy the weight loss benefits of cinnamon all day long.

2 cinnamon sticks
water
honey

In a kettle or saucepan of water, add cinnamon sticks broken into two and bring water and sticks to a boil. Allow to boil for a few minutes and then remove from heat. Let cinnamon tea steep for 5 additional minutes. Pour a cup into your favorite teacup and add a teaspoon of honey.

Cinnamon Lemonade

Here is a refreshing cinnamon lemonade for warm summer days.

2 quarts of water
3/4 cups sugar
3 cinnamon sticks
1 cup lemon juice
1 tsp whole cloves
Fresh lemon slices

Combine water, sugar, cinnamon sticks and cloves in a small pot on medium heat. Bring to a boil. Reduce heat and simmer for 20 minutes. Remove from heat and pick out cinnamon sticks and cloves. Pour into a pitcher and add lemon juice and lemon wedges. Refrigerate for at least two hours before serving.

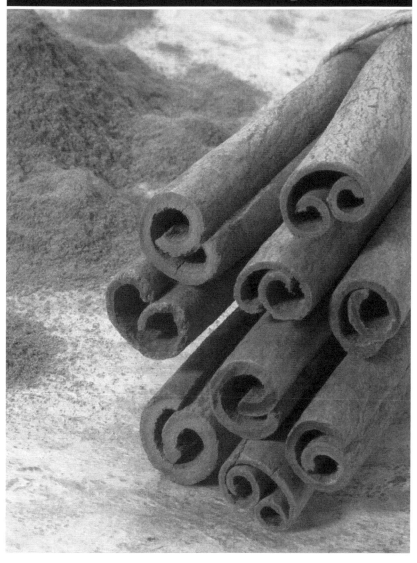

CHAPTER TEN
A Few of the Best Recipes Ever

Making cinnamon part of your health regimen doesn't have to be complicated...or boring! Cinnamon can be made a part of your life easily and deliciously!

Ready for some scrumptious ways to incorporate cinnamon into your daily diet? Try a few of these mouthwatering ideas today!

Yes! Cinnamon chips are made with a delicious blend of cinnamon and chocolate in a small chip formation which makes them excellent for baking (and snacking!). What a delicious way to incorporate cinnamon into your diet!

Not only will we learn some of the best cinnamon recipes ever, but why not try a few simple ways to enjoy the wonderful taste of cinnamon that are quick, easy and at your fingertips! You can try:

- Sprinkle cinnamon on your morning applesauce.

- Swirl a cinnamon stick into your favorite tea or coffee.

- Try a snack of peanut butter on cut apple wedges with a light sprinkling of cinnamon.

- Cinnamon on steak? Of course! In many cultures throughout the world, cinnamon is used to spice up a savory steak or other fine meats.

- Use a little cinnamon powder in your morning oatmeal

- Make a delicious spread consisting of honey and a little cinnamon to spread on a bagel or slice of toast.

In considering cinnamon as an accompaniment to dishes, our minds most often travel to rich desserts or amazing breads. And while desserts and breads are well deserving of cinnamon's attention, masterful dishes of both entrees and sides can be equally delightful.

Savory meats, delicate vegetables, and even fish and fruit can be the basis for wonderful cinnamon delicacies. Let your imagination run wild as you discover for yourself what cinnamon can do for sweet and savory dishes alike.

A few foods you may wish to add the flavor of a touch of cinnamon include:

Fish

- Cinnamon awakens taste buds for no more bland fish dishes.

- Cod

- Perch – spice before cooking

- Haddock

- Fish sticks

- Dipping sauce for frozen fish, breaded or battered

Meats

- In Medieval times cinnamon was used to help preserve meat – but more importantly it was used to cover up the odor and taste of meat that was slightly rotted.

- Today, cinnamon is frequently used in curry. Beef curry in particular needs cinnamon to be at its best.

- Moroccan's make a traditional stew with chickpeas, lentils, lamb, tomatoes, thin noodles, beaten eggs and, of course, cinnamon.

- In Sicily, ricotta cheese, sweetened and seasoned with cinnamon is considered extra special filling for ravioli.

- Add half a teaspoon cinnamon to chili. Also a good addition to vegetable soup.

- Add a couple of teaspoons of cinnamon to any commercial meat rub.

- Cinnamon is an excellent accompaniment to pork entrees, either sprinkled on the pork itself, or served within a delicious side dish of cinnamon apple raisins (recipe can be found in this book).

- Try cinnamon mixed in with rice and served with cut up portions of beef.

- Chicken has long been served as both a sweet and savory dish. Try adding a little cinnamon flavor to sweet chicken served in oriental dishes or a quick sprinkle over kebabs.

- Make a wonderful duck salad with poached egg, cranberries, pecans, balsamic vinegar and a touch of cinnamon for a delectable gourmet entree.

- Enjoy the rustic flavors of savory chili by adding cinnamon to your favorite stews and ground beef chili.

- Try serving little meatballs in spicy sauce, on toothpicks with several dipping sauces, including mustard and cinnamon.

- Add a touch of cinnamon to venison to further enhance its rustic flavor.

- Quail is a favorite to add a little cinnamon to for a spicy treat.

- Do you make home made jerky? You MUST use a little cinnamon on that jerky for an extra special savory treat.

Eat Your Veggies

Cinnamon on your veggies? Absolutely! Cinnamon enlivens bright colored veggies. Be sure to incorporate cinnamon on any of these wonderful vegetables for a full flavor dish.

You can not only add cinnamon directly to the vegetables themselves, but it is also an excellent choice for spicing up cream vegetable sauces, particularly around the holidays. And don't forget — add a quick splash of vinegar added to the cinnamon cream sauce to wake up the flavors nicely.

- Broccoli
- Cauliflower
- Celery

- Carrots
- Squash
- Zucchini
- Green beans
- Corn
- Peas

Root Vegetables

Root vegetables benefit amazingly from cinnamon's crisp flavor.

- Potato cakes
- Polenta
- Rice
- Turnips

Soups

- Sweet potato
- Gumbo
- Jamaican
- Caribbean
- Cold soups; add a few floating raisins and a dab of sour cream

Fruit Dishes

- Apple
- Blueberry
- Pineapple
- Oranges
- Strawberries
- Cherry crisp

- Papaya
- Grapefruit salad

Breads

- Cinnamon bread
- Cinnamon raisin bread
-

Cookies

- Thin cinnamon crisps
- Oatmeal
- Sugar
- Nut balls
- Date rolls

Cakes

- Sauce over sponge cake
- Spice cake

Pies

- Pecan

Puddings and Custards

- Rice
- Bread
- Chocolate bread
- Creamy chocolate cinnamon
- Egg custard
- Sauce over sponge cake
- Creme brulee

Recipes

Cinnamon is a fantastic spice for use in sweet or savory dishes. In fact, it is a wonderful accompaniment for salty foods such as honeyed nuts and even beverages. Enjoy these recipes as you discover for yourself the unique yet familiar flavor cinnamon has to offer. In addition to the recipes you will find in this section, you may also want to check out a few of the low fat cinnamon recipes in the Cinnamon for Weight Loss chapter of this book.

BREAKFAST

Cinnamon French toast

Start your day off with homemade cinnamon toast.

1 egg
1/2 cup milk
1 tsp ground cinnamon
pinch of nutmeg
bread slices

Whisk egg and add milk. Blend together adding ground cinnamon and nutmeg. Heat a frying pan or griddle and spray with a light coating of cooking oil. Dip slices of bread into egg and cinnamon bath getting both sides coated. Cook on medium heat on griddle.

Cinnamon toast

1/4 cup sugar
1 tbsp cinnamon

Mix both ingredients together to use on buttered toast for a great, easy cinnamon toast.

Main Dishes

Best Southwest Burgers

Here's a recipe that's sure to get rave reviews at your next barbecue.

   1 lb ground beef
   1 egg, slightly beaten
   1/2 tsp garlic salt
   1/4 tsp cinnamon
   1/8 tsp cayenne pepper

Combine all ingredients in a bowl and mix thoroughly. Form hamburgers and cook over grill until desired doneness. Why not serve this with a batch of sweet potato fries?

Magnificent Meatloaf

This recipe for meatloaf is sure to be a crowd pleaser!

   1 lb ground beef
   1 egg, slightly beaten
   1 onion, finely chopped
   1 celery stalk, finely chopped
   1/4 red pepper, finely chopped
   1 cup seasoned bread crumbs
   1 tbsp Worcestershire sauce
   3 tbsp tomato paste
   1/2 tsp garlic salt
   1/4 tsp cinnamon
   1/4 tsp cayenne pepper
   1/2 cup favorite pasta sauce

Mix all ingredients together. Place in loaf pan and bake at 350° for one hour, or until done.

Cincinnati Chili

Be sure to add this famous chili to your home recipe collection. It's a show stopper and great for holiday parties or game-day celebrations! Cincinnati Chili is even better if cooked a day ahead of time, and then allowed to sit in the refrigerator overnight until all of the flavors have blended together.

    1 pound ground beef
    1 tbsp vegetable oil
    1 vidalia onion, finely chopped
    2 cloves garlic, minced
    2 tbsp chili powder
    1 tsp ground cinnamon
    1 tsp ground cumin
    1 tsp ground allspice
    1/2 tsp salt
    1/2 tsp cayenne pepper
    1/4 tsp paprika
    1 oz unsweetened chocolate
    1 tbsp Worcestershire sauce
    1 (15-ounce) can of your favorite tomato sauce
    1 tbsp apple cider vinegar
    1/2 cup water
    1 (16-ounce) package uncooked spaghetti
    1/2 cup shredded cheddar cheese
    sour cream

Heat vegetable oil over medium heat. Add chopped onion and cook, stirring often, until tender; about 5 minutes. Add ground beef and continue cooking until beef is cooked all the way through.

Add all ingredients except pasta, cheddar cheese and sour cream. Stir and combine well. Continue cooking over low heat for 1 -2 hours, until flavors have a chance to meld together. For most robust flavor, spoon chili into a bowl and store covered in the refrigerator overnight.

When ready to serve, reheat chili on medium heat until warmed throughout. Serve over cooked spaghetti and top with shredded cheddar cheese. Add a dollop of sour cream, if desired.

Sweet Chicken Kebabs
This is a pretty entree that can either be cooked over the grill, or broiled in the oven. Just make sure chicken is cooked all the way through before serving.

> 1 lb boneless chicken breasts, in large cubes or strips
> pineapple, chunked
> cherry tomatoes, whole
> green pepper, cut into 1-1/2" strips
> 1/2 cup honey
> 1/2 tsp cinnamon
> wooden skewers

Combine honey and cinnamon in a small bowl and set aside. On wooden skewers, alternate threading chicken, pineapple, tomato and pepper (and repeat), leaving about one inch on each end for gripping.

Brush on honey cinnamon mixture and broil or grill until chicken is cooked throughout.

Serve hot with warm cinnamon rice.

Cinnamon Beef and Squash

Cinnamon is not just for dessert. It can be an excellent addition to savory entrees.

Cooked beef cubes
1 1/2 cup squash, cubed
1 tsp cinnamon
1/4 tsp paprika
2 tbsp butter, melted
1 small jar chopped mushrooms
2 garlic cloves, minced
1 tbsp chopped onion
2 tbsp cilantro, chopped
1 tbsp parsley, chopped
1/4 tsp salt
olive oil

In a large saucepan, heat a few tablespoons of olive oil over medium heat. Add onion and garlic and cook for 2 minutes. Add cubed squash and cook, stirring often, until squash is almost tender but still slightly firm. Add cooked squash and onion along with cooked beef cubes, mushrooms, cinnamon, paprika, melted butter, cilantro, parsley and salt. Stir all ingredients together and cook until hot throughout over medium heat.

Serve warm with cinnamon rice.

Side Dishes

Cinnamon Rice

Try this cinnamon rice recipe for a special accompaniment with your next special dinner. Guests will love it.

> 1 cup uncooked rice
> 2 cup water
> 2 tsp butter
> pinch of salt
> 1 tsp sugar
> 3/4 tsp cinnamon
> pinch of cloves

In a medium saucepan, add water, rice, butter and salt and bring to a boil over medium high heat. While waiting to boil, combine sugar, cinnamon and cloves in a small dish, and set aside. After mixture comes to a boil, turn heat down to a simmer and cover pan. Continue cooking 15 to 20 minutes until water is full absorbed. Fluff rice with a fork and sprinkle with cinnamon clove mixture. Serve warm.

For a special addition, consider adding raisins or slivered almonds to your rice dish.

Potato Salad

Here is a new twist on an old favorite. Add a little cinnamon to your next picnic's potato salad.

6 medium potatoes, cooked and cubed
1 cup mayonnaise
1 tbsp sugar
1 tbsp apple cider vinegar
2 tsp yellow mustard
3/4 tsp salt
3/4 tsp garlic powder
1/2 tsp ground cinnamon
1/2 tsp ground pepper
1/2 cup onion
2 celery stalks, finely chopped
4 eggs, hard boiled, cubed
paprika

Place boiled, cubed potatoes in a large bowl. In a separate bowl, combine mayonnaise, sugar, vinegar, mustard, salt, garlic powder and pepper. In another bowl, mix together onion, chopped celery and eggs. Combine egg mixture with mayonnaise mixture and mix well. Add to cubed potatoes and thoroughly combine. Chill in refrigerator for about 30 minutes. Season lightly with paprika.

Sweet Potato Fries

Try this recipe for a great twist on already amazing sweet potato fries.

    4 sweet potatoes
    cinnamon
    cayenne pepper
    salt
    vegetable oil, if desired

Peel sweet potatoes and cut into fries with a French fry chopper or by hand. Sprinkle fries with cinnamon and a little cayenne pepper. Add a bit of salt.

Either bake fries in oven at 400° until crispy (about 20 minutes), or deep fry in vegetable oil.

Cinnamon Raisin Apples

Try this southern side dish with your next family dinner, and enjoy all the raves!

    3 tart apples (Granny Smith and Fuji work great)
    1/4 cup raisins
    1/2 tsp cinnamon
    pinch of nutmeg
    2-3 tbsp butter

Peel and core apples, and slice into 1/4" wedges. Melt butter in a medium saucepan. Add apples and cook 2-3 minutes. Add raisins, cinnamon and nutmeg. Continue cooking until apples are tender and raisins are plump. Serve warm.

Cinnamon apple raisins are the perfect accompaniment to pork and beef entrees and beef, and as an ice cream topping.

DESSERTS

Apple Cinnamon Crepes

Enjoy this delicious crepe recipe with cinnamon apples as the star ingredients.

1 egg
1/2 cup flour
4 tbsp milk
pinch salt
3 tbsp sugar
1 tsp cinnamon
1 large tart apple (Granny Smith and Fuji work well)
2 tbsp butter
cooking spray or vegetable oil
Whipped cream

Whisk egg until smooth, then add milk, flour, and salt. Spray griddle or crepe pan with cooking spray or coat a thin coat of vegetable oil. Pour a thin layer of crepe batter in a circular shape and cook over medium-high heat until light bubbles begin to form in the crepe. Flip crepe and cook on opposite side until crepe is a very light golden color. Repeat process until crepe batter is used up. Place crepes on a warming tray or store in a warm oven or microwave until filling is complete.

Peel, core and slice apples into 1/8" slices. Melt 2 tablespoons of butter in a medium saucepan. Add apples, sugar and cinnamon. Cook apples and sugar cinnamon mixture until apples are tender. Remove from heat.

Place one crepe on a plate and add a few tablespoons of filling to the center of crepe. Fold over edges and serve warm with whipped cream, if desired.

Luscious Ice Cream Topping

Short on time, but need an amazing dessert to serve guests? Give this cold dessert a try.

1 tsp cinnamon
1/4 tsp nutmeg
1 tbsp dark brown sugar
Vanilla ice cream
Walnuts or pecans, chopped

Combine cinnamon, nutmeg and brown sugar and sprinkle over scoops of vanilla ice cream. For a crunchy treat, add 1 tablespoon of chopped pecans or walnuts to the cinnamon mixture. Top with a whole nut. Beautiful, easy and delicious!

Honey Cinnamon Topping

This is a great topping for use on ice cream or pound cake. Or, use as a gourmet topping to liven up a plain cheesecake.

1/4 cup honey
1 tsp cinnamon
1/4 tsp nutmeg
1 tbsp butter
1 tbsp brown sugar
1/4 cup pecans

Over medium low heat, melt butter. Add honey, and brown sugar and combine thoroughly. Add cinnamon, nutmeg and pecans and heat throughout.

Serve topping warm.

Snickerdoodle Cookies

Here is a time-tested cinnamon cookie recipe passed down from generations to enjoy.

1 1/2 cups sugar
1/2 cup butter, softened
1/2 cup shortening
2 eggs
2 1/2 cups flour
1 tsp baking soda
1/2 tsp salt
2 tsp cream of tartar
1/3 cup sugar
1 tbsp cinnamon

In a mixing bowl, cream together butter, shortening and 1 1/2 cups of sugar. Add eggs one at a time. In a small bowl, combine flour, baking soda, salt and cream of tartar. Add dry flour ingredients to butter and egg mixture and combine. Roll dough into 1" balls. If dough is too sticky to roll, cover with plastic wrap and place in refrigerator for one hour.

Once balls have been made, make coating. Combine 1/3 cup of sugar with cinnamon. Carefully roll each ball in cinnamon coating and place 2" apart on an ungreased cookie sheet. Bake in preheated oven at 400° for 8-10 minutes until done.

Cinnamon Cookies

Whip up a batch of warm cinnamon cookies for your children or grandchildren. Take note, the sugar and cinnamon amounts of this recipe are divided and used in two different portions of the recipe. It might be helpful to read through the recipe's entire directions before beginning to bake.

1 cup plus 3 tbsp sugar, divided
2 tsp plus 1 tsp cinnamon, divided
1/2 cup butter, softened
1 egg
1/4 cup walnuts
1 tsp vanilla
pinch nutmeg
1 1/3 cup flour
1 tsp baking powder
1/4 tsp salt

In a small dish, combine 3 tablespoons sugar with 1 teaspoon cinnamon and set aside for later. This will be used as a coating for the cookies just before baking.

In a mixing bowl, cream butter, eggs, 1 cup sugar and vanilla. In another bowl, combine dry ingredients including 1 teaspoon cinnamon, nutmeg, flour, baking powder and salt. Add dry ingredients to creamed butter mixture. Stir in walnuts. Form dough into large ball and wrap in plastic wrap or cover; refrigerate for one hour.

Remove dough from refrigerator and roll dough into 1" balls. Roll each ball in cinnamon sugar mixture that was set aside earlier. Place each cookie 2" apart on parchment lined or lightly greased baking sheet. Bake at 350° for 8-10 minutes until just set.

Texas Sheet Cake

This new twist on an old classic is guaranteed to get rave reviews.

2 cups flour
2 cups sugar
1/2 cup butter, softened
1/2 cup oil
1 cup water
1/3 cup cocoa
2 eggs
2 tsp cinnamon
1 tsp vanilla
1 tsp baking soda
1/2 cup buttermilk
Texas Sheet Cake frosting, just prepared and still warm

In a small bowl, combine flour and sugar. Set aside. Place butter, cocoa, oil and water in a medium saucepan and turn the heat to medium high. Bring to a boil, and then gently pour hot butter mixture into same bowl as flour mixture. Combine thoroughly and add eggs. Now add cinnamon, baking soda and vanilla and stir together.

Pour completed cake batter into an ungreased 16" x 13" jelly roll pan. Bake for 18 to 20 minutes at 350° until cake springs back when gently touched in the center. Take out of the oven and immediately frost with Texas Sheet Cake Frosting (recipe below).

Texas Sheet Cake Frosting

Use this special frosting with the above Texas Sheet Cake recipe. Unlike most frostings, Texas Sheet Cake Frosting is poured over the cake as soon as it comes out of the oven, and before it has a chance to cool. Make sure to cook this frosting while the sheet cake is still baking in the oven, so it is ready when the cake has completed baking.

1/3 cup milk
1/2 cup butter
1/3 cup cocoa
2 cups confectioner's sugar
1 tsp vanilla
1 cup pecans, chopped (if desired)

In a small saucepan, heat milk, butter and cocoa, bringing to a boil. Transfer hot milk mixture to a mixing bowl. Add confectioner's sugar and vanilla and thoroughly combine until frosting is a smooth consistency and confectioner's sugar is no longer lumpy.

Pour over hot Texas Sheet Cake reaching all edges. Sprinkle pecans over cake.

Cinnamon Chocolate Fudge

Cinnamon serves as a delightful spice to turn ordinary chocolate fudge into a special confectionery treat.

- 1 can sweetened condensed milk
- 1 bag semi-sweet chocolate chips
- 1 tsp vanilla
- 1 tbsp cinnamon
- 2 tbsp unsalted butter

Line an 8" square baking dish with aluminum foil. Grease with butter and set aside.

Using a double boiler, melt chocolate chips until smooth. Stir in sweetened condensed milk, vanilla and cinnamon. Remove from heat and add unsalted butter. Beat with a wooden spoon or rubber spatula until fudge has thickened and all chips have melted.

Use a rubber spatula to pour fudge into prepared baking dish. Place in the refrigerator, cool and allow to set for 2 to 4 hours. Remove pan from refrigerator and place on counter top. Carefully use the edges of the foil to remove fudge, still in the foil, from baking dish. Peel back edges of foil and cut fudge into one inch squares.

Serve and enjoy.

Cinnamon Lollipops

Looking for a fun treat for children? Try these fun cinnamon lollipops. Be sure and visit your nearest baking store to pick up fun shaped candy molds to make the lollipops in.

These cinnamon lollipops are also ideal for treating a nagging cough or easing painful sore throat pain.

    1 cup sugar
    1/3 cup water
    1/4 cup light corn syrup
    1/4 tsp salt
    Cinnamon oil
    5 or 6 drops of red food coloring
    Candy molds
    Candy sticks
    Cooking spray

Lightly coat molds with cooking spray.

In a medium saucepan, combine sugar, water, corn syrup and salt. Cook over medium high heat, stirring constantly until syrup mixture comes to a boil. Stop stirring, but continue boiling until mixture reaches hard crack stage*. Remove from heat and add several drops of cinnamon oil and red food coloring.

Carefully pour liquid candy into prepared molds. Add sticks and allow to cool on the counter until candy reaches room temperature and hardens. Once candy has hardened, pop each lollipop out of its tray and wrap in plastic wrap.

*See Hard Crack Stage on next page

Cinnamon "Glass" Candy

This recipe for cinnamon glass candy makes a beautiful Christmas gift when packaged in glass decanters. It's also a delicious way to treat a nagging sore throat or cough.

2 1/2 cups white sugar
1 cup light corn syrup
1 cup water
2 tsp cinnamon oil
1 tsp red food coloring
Confectioner's sugar for dusting

Before beginning, dust a cookie tray with a thick coating of confectioner's sugar and put aside.

In a medium pot, cook corn syrup and sugar over medium-high heat. Continue stirring until sugar is completely dissolved into the corn syrup. Allow mixture to reach a boiling point and continue to boil until syrup reaches the hard crack stage* at about 300° F when tested with a candy thermometer. Remove syrup mixture from burner and add food coloring and cinnamon oil.

Pour cinnamon syrup onto prepared cookie sheet and allow to cool completely. Once cool, break candy into random sizes and shapes, and dust with additional confectioner's sugar. Candy must be coated in confectioner's sugar so pieces will not stick together when storing.

*Hard crack stage occurs when syrup reaches between 300° and 310° F when tested using a candy thermometer. You can also check the syrup without the use of a thermometer. Fill a glass with very cold or ice water. Take

*a bit of the cinnamon candy syrup on a spoon and allow
to drip into the water. If the syrup stays soft, it is not ready.
If the mixture forms into brittle threads upon coming into
contact with the water, it has reached the hard crack stage.*

SNACKS

Cinnamon Crisps
Try these for a wonderful, tasty treat.

    2 tortillas
    1 tbsp butter or margarine
    1 tbsp sugar
    1/2 tsp cinnamon

Combine cinnamon and sugar in a small bowl. Butter
tortillas and cut into wedges. Sprinkle with cinnamon sugar
mixture and bake in oven at 350° for 10 to 12 minutes, or
until crispy.

Tasty Honeyed Nuts
Make a batch or two of these honeyed nuts for a healthy
evening snack.

    2 cups of your favorite nuts
    1/3 cup honey
    1 tsp cinnamon

In a bowl, combine all ingredients, gently stirring until nuts
are thoroughly coated in honey and cinnamon. Spread
coated nuts on a baking sheet and bake for 20 minutes at
375°. Enjoy!

Cinnamon Honey Spread

This is an easy way to add and enjoy cinnamon in your regular diet. Make it fresh each morning, or triple the recipe and make a larger batch to enjoy throughout the week.

1 tbsp honey
1/4 tsp cinnamon

Mix both ingredients together and use as a spread on bagels, warm toast, or cinnamon raisin bread.

Beverages

In olden days, cinnamon was used to make a spiced wine known as Hippocras. Cinnamon enhances the taste of liquid refreshments. Not only does it taste good, it is a very healthy addition to a healthy diet.

Vanilla Smoothie

Here is another luscious drink to add to your beverage list for guests.

1/4 cup cinnamon schnapps
3/4 cup cream soda
1/2 tsp vanilla
1/4 tsp cinnamon
1 cup crushed ice

Combine top four ingredients together and then blend with 1 cup crushed ice and serve with a long handled spoon.

Creamy Cider

Have you been looking for the perfect fall drink to spice up the cool, crisp evenings? Try this one.

1/4 cup cinnamon schnapps
1/2 cup apple cider
1/4 cup vanilla ice cream
1/4 tsp cinnamon

Combine all ingredients in a blender and sprinkle the top with 1/4 teaspoon cinnamon.

Here are a few amazing non-alcoholic treats to keep in mind the next time you host a party or family event.

Spicy Cider Punch

This is the perfect fall punch to serve with dinner. For best results, visit your local apple orchard to find the freshest apple cider around.

1 quart apple cider
1 quart lemonade
1/2 cup dark brown sugar
1/4 tsp allspice
1/4 cup cloves
1 tsp cinnamon

Combine all ingredients together and allow to rest for about 20 minutes to combine all the flavors. Spicy cider punch can be served either ice cold, or warmed over the stove and served in a mug.

Pretty Party Punch

Here is a pretty punch to serve at your next fall party.

  1 quart apple cider
  1 quart lemonade
  2 cups orange juice
  1/2 cup dark brown sugar
  1/4 tsp allspice
  1/4 cup cloves
  1 tsp cinnamon

Mix all the ingredients together and pour into a pretty punch bowl. Float very thin slices of lemons and oranges in the punch.

Tangy Citrus Punch

Here is another pretty party punch for you and your friends to enjoy.

  1 quart unsweetened grapefruit juice
  1 quart lemonade
  1 quart orange juice
  1/2 cup light brown sugar
  3 tsp cinnamon
  1/2 tsp nutmeg
  1 tsp cloves
  1 cup chopped oranges and grapefruit segments
  I tablespoon orange zest
  Maraschino cherries

Mix all ingredients well and add a handful of Maraschino cherries to complete this tangy treat. Best if permitted to chill for two hours before serving.

Cinnamon Tea

Keep this healthful cinnamon tea recipe in mind at the first sign of cold or flu, or just to enjoy on a crisp fall day.

    1 cup boiling water
    1 tea bag containing your favorite black tea
    1 cinnamon stick
    1-2 tsp honey

Place cinnamon stick in your favorite tea cup and pour boiling water over stick. Allow to steep for 5 to 10 minutes, stirring the stick occasionally. Add your favorite tea bag and continue to steep an additional 2 or 3 minutes. Sweeten with all natural honey to taste. Enjoy.

To ensure your tea remains warm, you may wish to cover your teacup with a piece of plastic or cloth while allowing it to steep.

Chai Tea

Try this classic recipe for a warm chair tea in the winter months, or a cold summer treat served over ice.

    Black tea
    2 cups water
    2 cups whole or 2% milk
    1 tsp ground cinnamon
    1/2 tsp ground black pepper
    1/4 tsp ground ginger
    1/2 tsp ground cloves
    Pinch of cardamom

Combine all ingredients in a small pot. Heat over medium heat until hot throughout.

Apple Delight

Try this beverage to serve special friends or family.

    3 oz cinnamon schnapps
    3 oz orange juice
    3/4 cup applesauce
    1/2 tsp cinnamon
    1/2 cup crushed ice

Mix all ingredients for 30 seconds in a blender and serve in a tall glass.

Cranberry Surprise

Cranberry surprise is a wonderful drink to serve as part of a holiday celebration.

    3 oz cinnamon schnapps
    1/2 cup ginger ale
    1/2 cup cranberry juice
    1/4 tsp cinnamon

Combine all ingredients and serve over a tall glass of crushed ice.

Best Hot Chocolate

Try this quick and simple hot chocolate recipe on a cold winter night.

    1 cup hot chocolate
    1/4 tsp cinnamon
    1/4 tsp nutmeg

Mix well and top with a dab of whipped cream.

Double Rich Hot Chocolate

You'll find this gourmet hot chocolate recipe is well worth the extra steps involved in making it!

    1/4 cup cocoa
    1/4 cup brown sugar
    1 tsp cinnamon
    1 cup milk (or half and half)
    1 tsp vanilla

Gently warm milk or half and half over medium heat on the stove. Cook until tiny bubbles form around edges of pan, but do not allow to boil. Take care not to burn or scald milk. Remove from heat. Blend cocoa, brown sugar and cinnamon together and stir into hot milk. Add the vanilla and sip slowly.

Sweet Pineapple Juice

Make a glass or two of this pepped up pineapple juice to begin your morning.

    1 cup pineapple juice
    1 tbsp brown sugar
    1/2 tsp cinnamon

Combine all ingredients in a tall glass. Serve warm or cold with a sprinkle of cinnamon on top. For a pretty and tasty addition, roll a small piece of pineapple in brown sugar and sprinkle it with cinnamon. Make a small slit in the pineapple chunk and put it on the rim of your glass or cup.

Spruced-up Cinnamon Cola

Here is a simple way to spruce up boring cola.

    1/2 tsp cinnamon
    Crushed ice
    Cola

Fill a glass 3/4 full with crushed ice. Add cinnamon, then fill the glass with your favorite cola. Stir well to thoroughly mix the cinnamon throughout. Savor the flavor.

Better Apple Juice

Tired of the same old apple juice? Here is an easy fix to try!

Add 1/4 teaspoon cinnamon to apple juice to wake up and intensify its flavor.

Banana-Apple Delight

This is a great summer drink packed with nutrition.

    1 large banana
    1 cup apple juice
    1/4 cup brown sugar
    1/4 cup ground nuts
    1 tsp cinnamon

Mash the banana with the brown sugar and cinnamon. Combine banana mixture with apple juice in a blender on medium speed. Serve immediately in a wide glass.

For a slightly more tart flavor, cider may be substituted for apple juice.

CHAPTER ELEVEN
The World's Favorite: Cinnamon Buns

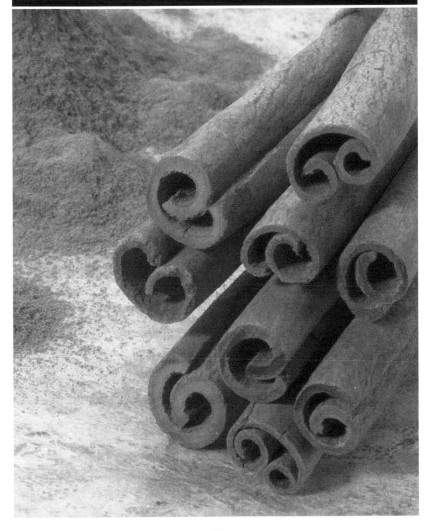

I know what you thought when you read the title of this chapter! "An entire chapter on cinnamon buns?"

That's right. An entire chapter on cinnamon buns. An entire chapter on those wonderful, warm, gooey breakfast treats we all can't wait to get our hands on.

Who doesn't like cinnamon buns? These treats are not just for breakfast pleasure any more. In fact, grandmother's cinnamon buns have become so wildly popular there is even a store located in many malls dedicated solely to selling cinnamon buns. This multi-million dollar confection industry has swept other markets as well, capitalizing on the comforting taste and smell of cinnamon in all its glory.

And, the cinnamon bun flavor and concept has wound up in some very unusual places. Did you know you can find the cinnamon bun flavor of choice in:

- Candles
- Lip gloss
- Essential oils
- Scented sprays
- Shampoos
- Shower gels
- Jewelry
- Cologne
- Lotions

At one time, cinnamon buns were even jointly packaged with comic books even further capitalizing on the popularity of the market.

But, while the cinnamon bun market is growing ever so quickly in popularity and introducing new twists on the old sticky bun, for space sake this chapter will deal with those wonderful sticky treats we all have grown to love.

Cinnamon buns became most popular in the southern portion of the United States and has grown country-wide. While no one seems to be able to stake claim to inventing the very first cinnamon bun, although many believe the origin is Swedish, the use of cinnamon being used as a spice in baked goodies dates back generations. Cinnamon was used to liven up baked confections by our grandparents and before, much of which has evolved into the scrumptious, gooey breakfast delight we now know as cinnamon buns.

But cinnamon buns are not solely an American concept. Although no one can be certain where they originated, countries all over the world boast their own version of these sweet cinnamon treats.

Northern Europe refers to the cinnamon bun as a sweet roll.

Germany has its Franzbrotchen.

Norway is known for its cinnamon bun that is free from sugary frosting, but still remains sweet and gooey in the layering of how its baked. They are called, skillingsboller, or penny buns.

Sweden calls it kanelbulle, which literally means "cinnamon bun." Did you know October 4 is national Cinnamon Bun Day in Sweden?

Finland boasts its Korvapuusti, which is a cinnamon bun nearly 8 inches wide. In fact, Finland also makes a wonderful dessert out of cinnamon buns where the buns are all packed side by side in a round cake pan as they bake to swell together into a delicious cake.

For the most part, cinnamon buns are comprised of a yeast based dough which is allowed to rise, spread with a sugar and cinnamon mixture, and then folded or rolled into that all too familiar bun. Many times it is then drenched in a lovely confectioner's topping or icing for added sweetness. But over the years, the cinnamon bun has evolved from a simple, rolled breakfast treat to a sometimes much more complex, coveted baked dessert.

In this chapter you will be introduced to several cinnamon bun recipes ranging from the simple to the not-so-simple; from the casual to the elegant. Some are recipes for the familiar cinnamon "bun" shape you are accustomed to. Others in more of a cake form, or special dessert.

Enjoy examining and testing out these amazing new recipes. Feel free to use them as a springboard to developing your own unique recipes, catered to you and your families likes and dislikes.

A few baking hints
Here are a few helpful tips before we get started.

Some of the recipes are slow rise, yeast based recipes, while others are quick rise. Pay careful attention to the type of yeast required, as using the wrong yeast can have unwanted results.

While cinnamon, sugar and even raisins make fantastic additions to your cinnamon bun recipes, remember that adding cinnamon to the bread dough batter itself can ruin the yeast action and cause the dough not to rise. Keep the cinnamon and sugar mixture as an added part after the dough has been made. One should never incorporate cinnamon and extra sugar into the dough mixture itself, as this will deter the leavening agent from making the dough rise. The best way to add flavorful cinnamon and sugar to your cinnamon buns is after the dough has risen. You will want to carefully roll out your raised dough and add the cinnamon sugar mixture to the top of the dough before rolling it into the bun.

We have given you several different frosting recipes for your cinnamon buns, ranging from sweet confectioner's sugar based icings to cream cheese frostings. While the individual recipes make recommendations on which frosting is best to use, feel free to switch icings according to your taste. You may also consider trying a favorite recipe of your own, or experiment developing a personalized recipe for yourself.

In addition to the ingredients listed in each recipe, consider trying a few of these additions for a special gourmet touch to your cinnamon rolls:

- Raisins
- Walnuts
- Pecans
- Cherries

- Cranberries
- Currents
- Nutmeg
- Cardamom
- Allspice
- Lemon zest
- Orange zest
- Orange frosting
- Brown sugar
- Pumpkin
- Vanilla
- Chocolate
- Maple
- Figs
- Dates

Recipes

Enjoy exploring and discovering some wonderful cinnamon bun recipes from this collection. When you're finished, why not try inventing a few of your own using your own unique flavor combinations.

We begin below with basic cinnamon filling recipes, along with sweet confectioner's frosting and a special cream cheese icing. We have even given you a basic starter recipe for bun dough. You may want to begin with these until you feel confident about trying some of the more gourmet recipes throughout this chapter.

Enjoy these as fillings and frostings with the bun recipes that follow.

Basic cinnamon roll dough (yeast recipe)

Here is a basic recipe for making cinnamon rolls using slow rising yeast. Use this a basis for concocting your own cinnamon buns using any combination of additional flavors and additions.

 2 cups milk
 3/4 cup sugar
 2 packets dry yeast
 1 1/4 tsp salt
 1 stick butter, softened
 3 eggs
 4 tbsp warm water
 7 cups of flour, divided

Over medium heat, cook milk until tiny bubbles form around edges. Be careful not to burn. Pour milk into a medium sized bowl and add sugar. Stir gently to dissolve and cool. In another bowl, combine 3 cups of flour with the yeast. Once cool, add flour and yeast mixture to milk and allow to rise undisturbed for one hour.

Add eggs, butter and remaining flour and combine thoroughly. Mix dough with an electric mixer using dough hooks for 5 minutes, or knead by hand for 10 minutes. Allow to rest an additional 10 minutes before rolling out and using.

For most recipes, cinnamon roll dough bakes at 350°.

Basic Cinnamon Roll Dough (non-yeast recipe)

Here is a basic recipe for making cinnamon rolls using slow rising yeast.

2 1/4 cups flour
2 tbsp sugar
1 tsp baking soda
1 tsp baking powder
1/2 tsp salt
1 1/4 cups buttermilk
6 tbsp unsalted butter, melted

In a small bowl, add flour, sugar, baking soda, baking powder and salt. Mix together. Add buttermilk and melted butter and combine until a soft dough forms.

Use this quick dough as a basis for ready-made cinnamon roll treats.

Cinnamon Filling

This is a basic cinnamon filling recipe to be used with any bun dough recipe.

3/4 cup packed dark brown sugar
3 tbsp granulated sugar
1 tsp cinnamon
pinch salt
1 tsp unsalted butter

Gently melt butter over medium heat. Add brown sugar, white sugar, cinnamon and salt and stir together. Use this filling to sprinkle or spread on dough before rolling and baking.

Vanilla Frosting

This is a classic confectioners' vanilla frosting that can be drizzled over the top of warm, fresh from the oven cinnamon buns.

 1/4 cup butter
 1 pound confectioner's sugar
 3 tbsp milk
 1/4 tsp vanilla

Combine all ingredients in a blender until creamy throughout. Drizzle over the tops of warm cinnamon buns or use as a dipping sauce.

Cream Cheese Frosting

Cream cheese frosting always makes a wonderful, grown-up alternative to confectioners' vanilla frosting. Frost buns while they are still warm for an extra special treat.

 8 oz cream cheese
 1/2 cup butter
 1 tsp vanilla
 4 cups confectioner's sugar
 2 tbsp milk

Mix all ingredients together in a medium mixing bowl with a blender on medium speed until thoroughly combined. Spread over top of warm cinnamon buns for an amazing flavor.

Best Cinnamon Rolls Ever

Here is one of the best cinnamon rolls around, and sure to be a show-stopper at your next brunch. This recipe takes some time, and can be even started the day before. For fresh cinnamon rolls in the morning, put this recipe together the day prior, and save the very last baking step for morning.

6 cups flour
2 pkg dry yeast
1 1/2 cups milk
1/2 cups butter
1/2 cups sugar
1 tsp salt
3 eggs
3/4 cup sugar
1/2 cup butter, softened
1 tbsp cinnamon
1/2 tsp allspice
1 tsp flour
1/2 cup raisins
1/4 cup walnuts, chopped finely
olive oil
vanilla frosting

In a medium saucepan, heat milk, 1/2 cup of butter, 1/2 cup sugar and salt. Warm until butter is just melted, but do not boil or scald milk. Remove from heat. In a medium mixing bowl, combine half the flour and both packages of yeast.

Add milk mixture to flour and yeast. Add eggs and beat on medium speed for 2 or 3 minutes. Add remaining flour and combine. Using dough hooks, beat dough for 5 minutes on medium speed until smooth and elastic.

Use olive oil to grease bottom and sides of a metal bowl. Place dough in oiled bowl and cover with a kitchen towel. Allow to rise undisturbed for one hour, until dough almost doubles.

While dough is rising, make the cinnamon filling. In a small bowl, combine 3/4 cup of sugar, 1/2 cup softened butter, 1 tablespoon cinnamon, 1/2 teaspoon allspice and 1 teaspoon of flour.

When dough has finished rising, punch down and divide into two balls. Cover each ball and allow to rise for an additional 15 minutes. On a floured surface, roll out each ball of dough into a 6 x 10" rectangle. Cover each dough rectangle with equal amounts of the cinnamon filling. Sprinkle raisins and walnuts on top of filling and roll each rectangle into a roll and slice into 3/4" slices. Place each individual cinnamon roll on a greased cookie sheet and cover with plastic wrap. Place tray of rolls in the refrigerator and let rise for at least 2 hours. Rolls can also rest in refrigerator overnight.

Prior to cooking, allow take rolls out of refrigerator and place on counter top for 1 hour. Dough should rise significantly during this final rise. Place in preheated oven and bake at 375° for 20 minutes, or until very slightly golden brown.

Take out of oven and frost with vanilla frosting. Serve warm and enjoy!

Individual Cinnamon Roll Tartlets

This is a wonderful cinnamon roll recipe that will always come out deliciously gooey and fantastically beautiful!

1 cup milk
1/2 cup sugar
1 packet dry yeast
1/2 tsp salt
1/2 cup butter, softened and divided
2 eggs
2 tbsp warm water
3 1/2 cup flour
3/4 cup packed dark brown sugar
3 tbsp granulated sugar
1 tbsp cinnamon

Topping (to be placed on bottom of muffin tin)
3/4 cup packed dark brown sugar
3 tbsp granulated sugar
1 tbsp cinnamon
1/2 cup walnuts, finely chopped
pinch salt
1/4 cup unsalted butter, melted

Over medium heat, cook milk until tiny bubbles form around edges. Be careful not to burn. Pour milk into a medium sized bowl and add 1/2 cup of sugar. Stir gently to dissolve and cool. In another bowl, combine flour with the yeast. Once cool, add flour and yeast mixture to milk and allow to rise undisturbed for one hour.

Add eggs, 1/4 cup butter and combine thoroughly. Mix dough with an electric mixer using dough hooks for 5 minutes, or knead by hand for 10 minutes. Allow to rest an additional 10 minutes before rolling out into a 1/4" thick rectangle.

In a bowl, combine 1/4 cup butter with 3/4 cup brown sugar, 3 tbsp sugar and 1 tbsp cinnamon. Spread this mixture over rolled out dough and roll into tight jelly roll, making certain to seal edge when finished. Using a sharp knife, cut into 1" slices.

In a small bowl, combined unsalted butter, brown sugar, 3 tbsp sugar, cinnamon, pinch of salt and walnuts.

In a muffin tin, place 1 teaspoon melted butter, swirling around to coat each tin (use additional butter, if necessary). Add equal amounts of cinnamon walnut mixture to the bottom of each tin. Place one sliced cinnamon roll, cut side down, into each tin. Bake at 350° for about ten minutes until done. Carefully remove from oven and flip tin over to invert the roll, now ending up with gooey walnut mixture on the top of roll. Serve warm and enjoy!

Cinnamon Bun "Dips"
This is a fast and easy treat is a fun play off cinnamon buns.

  2 tortillas
  2 tbsp melted butter
  3 tbsp sugar
  1 tsp cinnamon
  Confectioner's vanilla frosting

Coat tortillas with butter using a pastry brush. Mix sugar and cinnamon in a small bowl and sprinkle liberally over tortilla. Using a pizza cutter, cut into wedges. Bake in oven at 350° for 5 to 8 minutes. Serve warm using frosting as a dip.

Cake Mix Cinnamon Rolls

Here's a quick cinnamon roll recipe when you might be short on buttermilk or baking powder.

 1 box yellow cake mix
 5 cups flour
 1 packet yeast
 2 1/2 cups warm water (about 120°)
 3/4 stick butter, melted
 1/2 cup brown sugar
 1 tsp cinnamon
 olive oil

In a mixing bowl, combine cake mix, flour, yeast and warm water. Mix until well blended and smooth. Continue to beat with dough hooks on a medium setting for 5 or 6 minutes.

Brush the bottom and sides of a metal bowl with olive oil. Place dough in oiled bowl and cover with a towel. Allow to rise undisturbed for one hour.

After one hour, remove dough and divide into two equal portions. Rest again an additional 5 – 10 minutes. On a lightly floured surface, roll out each portion of dough into an 8 x 16" rectangle, about 1/4" in thickness. Brush each section of dough with melted butter. Sprinkle brown sugar and cinnamon on each, and roll. Be sure to gentle seal shut the edge of the roll so it doesn't open during baking. Cut each roll into 1/2" slices and place on a baking sheet and allow to rise one more time, for 5 to 10 minutes, until noticeably raised.

Bake in oven at 400° for 12 minutes.

Quick and Easy Cinnamon Rolls

Use this quick and easy cinnamon roll recipe when you are low on time.

1 loaf refrigerated bread dough
3 tbsp melted butter
1 tsp cinnamon
2/3 cup brown sugar
1/2 cup walnuts, finely chopped
vanilla frosting recipe

Spread bread dough on a cookie sheet about 1/4" in thickness for form a rectangle 6" wide. In a small bowl, combine cinnamon, brown sugar and walnuts; set aside. Melt butter in microwave and brush on top of dough. Sprinkle cinnamon brown sugar mixture heavily all over buttered dough.

Roll dough up into a tight roll, beginning at the long edge. Using a sharp knife, cut roll into 3/4" slices. Place each slice onto a buttered baking sheet. Bake at 350° for 20 to 25 minutes. Frost with vanilla frosting and serve warm.

Simple Cinnamon Roll Croissants

Here's a great breakfast treat when there isn't time for a yeast bread recipe. Serve these beautiful cinnamon roll croissants in a cloth-lined bread basket for an extra special touch.

1 tube refrigerated croissants
3 tbsp melted butter
1 tsp cinnamon

pinch allspice
2/3 cup brown sugar

Spread each individual croissant on a cookie sheet. In a small bowl, combine cinnamon, brown sugar and set aside. Melt butter in microwave and brush on top of dough. Sprinkle cinnamon and brown sugar mixture heavily all over buttered croissant.

Roll up each piece of dough into a croissant, beginning at the long edge, and forming a point at the end. Slightly curve edges of croissants and place onto a buttered baking sheet. Bake at 350° for 20 to 25 minutes. Serve warm.

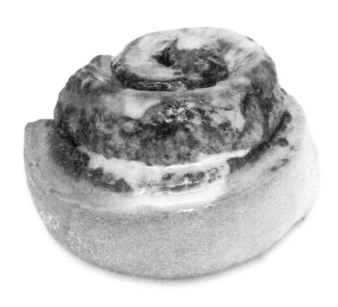

CHAPTER TWELVE
A Gentle Word of Caution

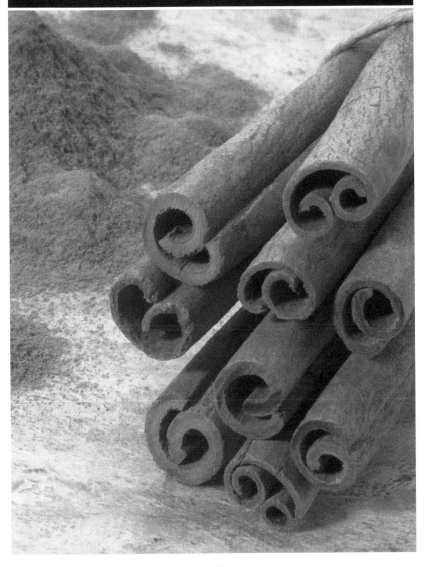

There is definitely truth to the saying there is "too much of a good thing." And cinnamon, just like most spices, herbs and any healing substance, is included. Before making regular use of any natural health or alternative treatment, talk openly and honestly with your own personal healthcare provider. Keep in mind this book is an attempt to share information. And as with any treatment, cinnamon has its limitations. Be sure to use it wisely and always in moderation. Pay close attention to any warnings listed throughout the book, and heed all cautions presented by your healthcare physician.

Every body is different. Just because a remedy works for one person, does not necessarily mean it will work for everyone. Our body chemistry is each different, as are the ways we react to natural health remedies.

In addition, be sure to be open with your physician about other medications you are taking, as well as conditions or illnesses you are struggling with. Cinnamon, like any herb, spice or medication, may react with other medications you are taking.

While there are more than one hundred types of cinnamon world wide, only two are popular in the United States. Cassia and Ceylon cinnamons are the most popular in this country, and can be found in both ground powder form and sold as a capsule. Cassia cinnamon contains higher levels of coumarin than Ceylon cinnamon, which can be dangerous in high levels for people struggling with liver disease. However, cinnamon sold in the United States is not required to divulge which type of cinnamon is being sold. Great care should be taken when adding cinnamon to a diet required to be free of coumarin. Be sure and consult your health care provider before staring any cinnamon regimen.

The information provided on these pages is intended as a record of folklore and is not intended as medical advice or for self-treatment. For medical problems, or before beginning diet modification, seek the advice of a qualified medical professional.

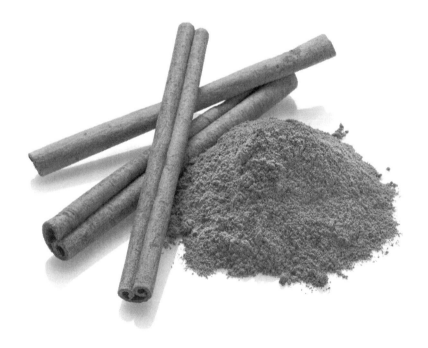

CHAPTER THIRTEEN
Frequently Asked Questions

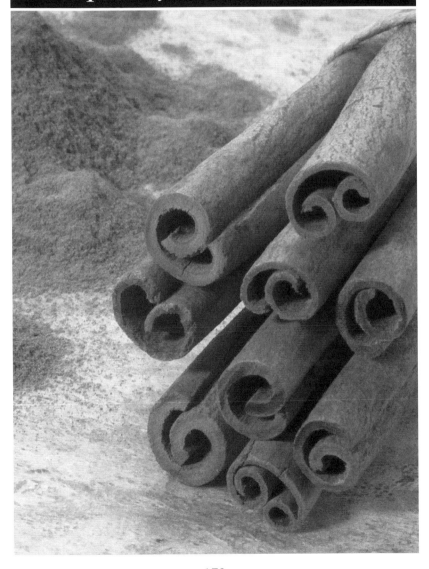

What is cassia? Is cassia cinnamon "true" cinnamon?
Cassia and "true" cinnamon are not the same thing. In most packaged "cinnamons," the cinnamon spice is really ground cassia, or a combination of ground cassia and ground cinnamon. Cassia, which is also in the cinnamon family, is actually a stronger spice than true cinnamon. So, we tend to use less of it than if we were purchasing true cinnamon.

True cinnamon is called Ceylon cinnamon. Most mass-produced cinnamons in the United States are the slightly inferior, cassia cinnamons.

What are cinnamon sticks?
Cinnamon sticks are actually the bark taken from evergreen trees. The bark is peeled from the trees and then allowed to dry. As the moisture is removed from the bark during the drying process, the bark naturally curls into its well-known cinnamon stick shape. **Can too much cinnamon be bad for me?**
Yes. There is such as thing as "too much of a good thing." Cassia cinnamon, which is the type of cinnamon most produced and available in the United States, can contain higher amounts of coumarin than true, purer Ceylon cinnamon.

People with liver problems, or who are taking drugs and medications that can over-tax the liver, should always consult their doctor before beginning any cinnamon use. Also, if you are diabetic or are taking drugs for blood thinning, cinnamon use should be monitored or avoided.

These side effects and warnings are geared toward cassia cinnamon. Ceylon cinnamon, which does not contain the volume of coumarin in that of cassia cinnamon, is considered safe. However, due to the fact that current packaging protocols in the United States do not require manufacturers to state which type of cinnamon is being used in the product, it is almost impossible to tell which type of cinnamon you are purchasing. Caution should be taken.

My supermarket only sells small containers of cinnamon. Where can I buy cinnamon in larger amounts or bulk quantities?

There are countless places to buy cinnamon in bulk. Try online or in many health food stores. Store managers can also order large, bulk containers of cinnamon for you.

How long does cinnamon last?

Like most spices, cinnamon's freshness is affected by sunlight, air and temperature. Stored properly, cinnamon can be expected to retain its freshness for long periods of time.

Ground cinnamon – 6 months for up to 2 years
Cinnamon sticks – 2 to 4 years

How do I best store cinnamon?

Cinnamon is best stored in a tightly sealed container, in a cool and dry, dark place. For ground or powdered cinnamon, store in a container with a tight fitting lid. Cinnamon sticks can easily be stored in a mason jar.

Can cinnamon sticks be re-used?

Cinnamon sticks are a great way to add flavor and spice to warm winter drinks. Feel free to use cinnamon sticks over and over again, to spice up a favorite cup of tea for instance, as long as the flavor allows. Just be sure to store the cinnamon stick safely being careful not to allow bacteria to develop.

What is the difference between cinnamon oil and cinnamon bark?

The biggest difference between cinnamon oil and cinnamon extract are the intensity of flavor, and the ability to withstand high heating temperatures.

Cinnamon oil is a highly concentrated form of cinnamon taken directly from the bark of cinnamon. Typically, cinnamon oil is four times as potent as its extract. Extract, a weaker form of cinnamon, is made by dissolving cinnamon or cinnamon oil in alcohol.

Cinnamon extract is an excellent choice for use in baked good, such as cakes, cookies, pies and even ice creams and sauces. Because of the high cooking temperatures associated with candy making, cinnamon oil is usually the best choice, as extracts tend to lose flavor at high temperatures.

Can I substitute cinnamon oil for cinnamon extract?

Cinnamon oil is a much stronger concentration than cinnamon extract. To substitute, replace 1 part cinnamon oil for 4 parts extract.

Does cinnamon retain its medicinal integrity after heating? Will cooking with cinnamon destroy any of its medicinal properties?

Most research studies conclude that cinnamon does not lose significant medicinal integrity through the heating process. So, whether you are enjoying cinnamon baked in bread, or sprinkling a little fresh cinnamon over your morning applesauce, you are still getting the full health benefits cinnamon has to offer!

My doctor has told me to watch coumarin intake. Should I still use cinnamon?

Cassia cinnamon contains higher levels of coumarin than Ceylon cinnamon. However, cinnamon sold in the United States is not required to divulge which type of cinnamon is being sold. Great care should be taken when adding cinnamon to a diet required to be free of coumarin. Be sure and consult your health care provider before staring any cinnamon regimin.

Where can I purchase Ceylon cinnamon?

In the United States, it can be very difficult to tell which type of cinnamon one is purchasing merely from looking on the package. While contacting the cinnamon manufacturer directly is an option, here are several references for purchasing Ceylon cinnamon on your own:

www.Penzys.com
www.ceylongcinnamon.com

How do I tell if the cinnamon sticks I am purchasing are the Ceylon or Cassia varieties? The package doesn't state.

While the FDA does not require the manufacturer to state which variety of cinnamon has been packaged, there are ways to help visually determine the type being purchased. Use the chart below to help determine which type of cinnamon you are using.

	Ceylon	Cassia
Color	Pale, tan, light color	Deep red rich color
Aroma	Lightly fragrant	Potent fragrance
Taste	Light, sweet flavor	Pungent taste
Cost	More expensive	Less expensive
Stick appearance	Dense centers, thin layers	More tubular, hollow, scrolls
Coumarin	.04% coumarin	5% coumarin

Where can I purchase Ceylon cinnamon capsules?

Cinnamon capsules can be purchased at most health food and nutrition stores, and can also be found in plenty on the Internet. Be sure to check the fine print if you are specifically wanting to purchase the Ceylon variety. The Ceylon variety of cinnamon capsules should be clearly marked. If not, when purchasing online contact the seller or manufacturer to be certain you are purchasing the desired variety.

What is organic cinnamon? Is there a difference?

Some harvesters of cinnamon have been known to treat cinnamon bark with a chemical solution during its drying period as a way of combating insects or infestation. While most reputable harvesters steer clear of this practice, it should be known that pretreating the drying bark can have negative effects on its ultimate quality. Organic cinnamon is usually guaranteed free of any pesticides or additives.

What are cinnamon chips? Are they made with real cinnamon?

Yes! Cinnamon chips are made with a delicious blend of cinnamon and chocolate in a small chip formation which makes them excellent for baking (and snacking!). What a delicious way to incorporate cinnamon into your diet!

Does cinnamon gum have any health benefit?

The University of Illinois at Chicago has conducted research concluding that cinnamon gums contain many of the same antibacterial properties as the cinnamon spice. This antibacterial property works to fight bacterial germs of the mouth and also combat bad breath.

What is the Cinnamon Challenge? Is it dangerous?

BEWARE! The Cinnamon Challenge is an extremely dangerous "dare" that has made its way in popularity on the Internet and throughout our schools. In this challenge, the user is challenged to swallow 1 full teaspoon of cinnamon, without water, in 60 seconds. While this may sound like a harmless teenage dare, the effects can be permanent and detrimental. Participants have suffered loss of consciousness, collapsed lungs, and even death.

The human body cannot consume and digest cinnamon without the aid of water. Cinnamon's tiny particles can obstruct airways in the lungs and in some cases cause the lung to collapse. Permanent scarring can occur and the use of a ventilator can be required to aid in breathing.

The Cinnamon Challenge is extremely dangerous and should never be taken.

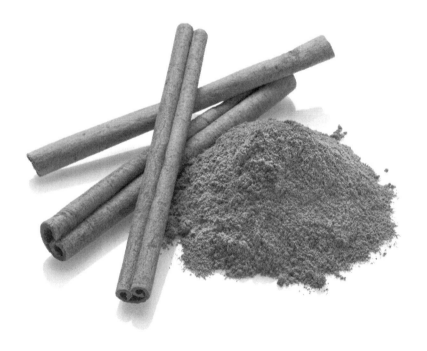

Additional books by Emily Thacker

Additional books by Emily Thacker
can be ordered using the attached order form
at the back of this book,
or by visiting our website at

http://www.jamesdirect.com

THE VINEGAR BOOK

Everyone loves vinegar! Its piquant bite blends well with an endless number of other foods. It tenderizes, enhances and preserves foods. More importantly, vinegar is a terrific germ killer. It is active against bacteria, viruses, molds and fungus. This safe, healing food can be found all across the world in many forms and flavors.

It is the traveler's friend, as it helps to prevent the system upsets that often plague tourists. Research has shown it to be effective in killing flu germs. It is also known for its anti-itch properties and its muscle soothing abilities.

Vinegar's long history as a panacea for the aches and pains of this world is respected in many cultures and places. Anyone who is serious about natural healing, old time remedies or folk medicine must have this book! (Also consider *THE VINEGAR ANNIVERSARY BOOK*, a blending of four separate books on vinegar: *THE VINEGAR BOOK, THE VINEGAR BOOK II, THE VINEGAR HOME GUIDE and THE VINEGAR DIET.*)

To find out more about *THE VINEGAR BOOK*, use the order form at the end of this book, or visit the publisher's website:

http://www.jamesdirect.com

THE VINEGAR BOOK II

This delightful addition to Emily Thacker's series of four books on vinegar takes you through the year, with a vinegar use for each day.

Twelve chapters, one for each month, combine the 365 vinegar based hints with explanations of how vinegar is made, why it is so healthful and how it has been used down through thousands of years.

You will learn of vinegar's uses in cooking and preserving and about its value is preventing diseases. This includes its importance in fighting cancer and arthritis, as well as how vinegar can be used to actually "cook" protein, such as fish.

This book also contains easy directions for making fruit, vegetable and herbal vinegars. You will see how to begin with apple cider vinegar and add rose petals to inspire love and romance, valerian as a sleep aid, bay leaves to sharpen the memory or gota kola to fight stress.

You will also find a recipe for making imitation balsamic vinegar that rivals the expensive varieties for taste and usefulness!

To find out more about *THE VINEGAR BOOK II*, use the order form at the end of this book, or visit the publisher's website:

http://www.jamesdirect.com

THE MAGIC OF HYDROGEN PEROXIDE

One of the most unusual books I have written, because it not only covers the healthy attributes of hydrogen peroxide but also talks about its use as an alternate fuel source. In these times of concern about running out of complex petroleum based fuels, hydrogen peroxide's simple formula and renewable attributes make it an important part of both today's energy production and tomorrow's energy needs.

In addition to being an excellent propellant, hydrogen peroxide has a long history of medicinal use. It is well know for its ability to cleanse and disinfect wounds. Less well known is its ability to disinfect water and sanitize many kinds of medical equipment.

Hydrogen peroxide is used to dissolve earwax and to prevent infection in scrapes and cuts. It is also part of some enjoyable, but safe, chemical experiments for children.

To buy an additional copy of *THE MAGIC OF HYDROGEN PEROXIDE*, use the order form at the end of this book, or visit the publisher's website:
http://www.jamesdirect.com

THE HONEY BOOK

Everyone loves the magical taste of honey! From the rumbly tumbly of Winnie the Pooh to your great grandmother's special home remedy for easing that nagging sore throat pain, honey has long been nature's "liquid gold."

Research studies have shown that honey possesses unique and remarkable nutrients that bring healing to the body effectively and naturally, without harmful side effects that occur with so many pharmaceutical medications. Honey is an all-natural, inexpensive and readily-available alternative to treat the body's ailments.

Honey contains powerful antibacterial and antimicrobial qualities that are effective in treating open cuts, wounds and bacterial infections. Honey is also excellent for treating fatigue, arthritis and joint pains, digestion problems and respiratory ailments — just to name a few!

Contained in *The Honey Book* are 208 pages of natural home remedies, research and recipes for putting honey to use immediately against some of your most bothersome health issues and conditions.

To find out more about *The Honey Book*, use the order form at the end of this book, or visit the publisher's website:
http://www.jamesdirect.com

GARLIC:
NATURE'S NATURAL COMPANION

This volume is a celebration of the miraculous healing powers of garlic! Across the world, it is used as a vegetable, a health food and to empower the immune system. Garlic has an almost endless number of aromatic compounds that constantly react with air and the foods it comes into contact with. These complex new mixtures produce the tantalizing aromas associated with this remarkable vegetable.

From earliest times garlic's ability to kill germs and heal sickness has been recognized. It has been used as an amulet to frighten away vampires and combined with vinegar to make the Thieves' Vinegar that reputedly offered protection from the plague.

Garlic grows almost everywhere, from the cold of Siberia and Tibet to the warmth of the Mediterranean and sunny California. Much of the world's supply is grown in China, who ships it out by the ton. It comes in tiny, intense, almost bitter bulbs to large elephant garlic bulbs.

The wonder of this versatile food is celebrated in festivals and fairs. Cook offs feature it in surprising recopies. Garlic is truly one of the healthiest, most widely used healing foods on the planet!

To find out more about *GARLIC: NATURE'S NATURAL COMPANION*, use the order form at the end of this book, or visit the publisher's website:
http://www.jamesdirect.com

THE MAGIC OF BAKING SODA

Do you keep your baking soda in the refrigerator or in the medicine cabinet? Or, perhaps you keep it with your laundry or cleaning supplies? Whether you call it bicarbonate of soda, sodium bicarbonate, bread soda … or plain old baking soda … this remarkable powder has hundreds of uses. You will want to keep it in your kitchen, medicine cabinet and with your cleaning and laundry supplies.

Baking soda is a naturally occurring substance that is kind to the environment. It is used to soothe allergies, exactly the opposite of many harsh chemical cleaning supplies. Most of the world's baking soda comes from a single huge deposit located in Wyoming.

Whether it is to soothe an acid stomach or the itching of rashes, baking soda is a must-have for the medicine cabinet. It is used in hospitals to protect the kidneys from intravenous dyes used in CT scans and to assist in dialysis treatments. Make sure you are getting all the benefits possible from this inexpensive substance you already have in your home.

To find out more about *THE MAGIC OF BAKING SODA*, use the order form at the end of this book, or visit the publisher's website:
http://www.jamesdirect.com

THE VINEGAR HOME GUIDE

Distilled or "white" vinegar is usually used for cleaning. Because white vinegar is a colorless liquid it is less likely to discolor articles being cleaned. This guide will show you when to clean with vinegar and when not to clean with vinegar.

Vinegar contains a host of germ fighting components it has both antibiotic and antiseptic properties. It has the ability to actually kill mold and mildew spores. And, it can contain natural tannins which help to preserve foods.

Vinegar is a completely biodegradable product nature can easily break it down into components that feed and nurture plant life. This makes it superior to chemical cleaners that poison the soil today and remain in it and destroy plant life for many years.

This helpful book is packed full of ways to use vinegar around the home, in the garden, on pets and to clean the car, boat or camper. You will want to use vinegar in your humidifier, to strip wallpaper, repair wood scratches kill mold on refrigerator and freezer gaskets and to make both play-clay and mouthwashes.

To find out more about *THE VINEGAR HOME GUIDE*, use the order form at the end of this book, or visit the publisher's website:
http://www.jamesdirect.com

VINEGAR & TEA

Green tea is both soothing to the body and healing for the spirit. Medical research continues to add to the long list of healing properties of green tea. It is a safe, tasty way to lose weight and improve health.

For many thousands of years tea has been used to improve health and vitality. Tea contains much less caffeine than stimulates such as coffee, and even more importantly, contains a different kind of caffeine. Scientific studies and detailed chemical analysis show that the type of caffeine in tea is less likely to cause the irritating, jittery symptoms of coffee and other caffeine containing substances. In fact, tea is often considered a soothing, calming liquid that brings a sense of well being and serenity.

The *Vinegar & Tea* book describes the way tea is pro-duced and grown and explains which kinds may be perfect for you. It covers delicate white teas, healing green ones and bold black blends. It will guide you in choosing the per-fect tea to heal illnesses or soothe a troubled spirit.

To find out more about *Vinegar & Tea*, use the order form at the end of this book, or visit the publisher's website:
http://www.jamesdirect.com

EMILY'S DISASTER GUIDE OF NATURAL REMEDIES

EMILY'S NEW GUIDE TO NATURAL TREATMENTS
FOR INFECTIOUS DISEASE

Our world is changing. Like it or not, in our post-September 11 world, we live under the threat of a terrorist strike. Hurricane Katrina has reminded us that nature can be brutal, with heavy consequences for those in nature's path or for citizens unprepared. Our increased mobility with air transportation means any disease outbreak, anywhere in the world, can be at our doorstep in mere days.

EMILY'S DISASTER GUIDE OF NATURAL REMEDIES is a unique guide written to highlight some of the many threats we face, both natural and man made, and ways to prepare and protect your family.

Included in this guide is an overview of current events and the state our communities are in. You will also find a list of infectious diseases and conditions, along with possible treatments.

PLUS each book contains its own Emergency Preparedness Checklist and Emergency Family Plan to help your family prepare for any emergency.

To find out more about *EMILY'S DISASTER GUIDE OF NATURAL REMEDIES*, use the order form at the end of this book, or visit the publisher's website:
http://www.jamesdirect.com

THE VINEGAR ANNIVERSARY BOOK

The Vinegar Anniversary Book blends the contents of Emily Thacker's four books on vinegar into one big book!

The original *Vinegar Book* details hundreds of old time healing remedies plus information on how to clean with vinegar. You will learn about the many different kinds of vinegar – from apple cider, wine, rice and malt to more exotic kinds such as banana and date.

The *Vinegar Book II* offers 365 vinegar uses to let you try a new one every day of the year.

The *Vinegar Home Guide* focuses on using vinegar for cleaning and disinfecting around the home, yard and garden.

The *Vinegar Diet Book* brings all the healthy goodness of vinegar to the table in an exciting, safe way to easily control weight. This remarkable way to manage weight offers wholesome, nourishing insight into managing what you eat. You will find this is the easiest, most foolproof diet plan you have ever tried!

To find out more about *The Vinegar Anniversary Book*, use the order form at the end of this book, or visit the publisher's website:

http://www.jamesdirect.com

Thank You!

Thank you, once again, dear reader, for your continued interest in natural healing ways. It has been a pleasure to bring you this book, and all its exciting uses for cinnamon.

If you have a natural healing remedy, unique or special cleaning method or an old-time recipe that your family has used, would you consider sharing it with other readers just like yourself? If I use it in one of my upcoming books, you will receive a free copy of the book upon printing.

Please fill out the form that follow and mail it back to me. If the form is missing or isn't available, feel free to use a sheet of paper and mail your ideas in to us.

Thank you again, and my warmest wishes for a long, healthy, happy life.

Emily Thacker

Emily, here is one of my favorite uses for cinnamon:

_____

_____

_____

_____

_____

_____

Can we use your name and city when crediting this remedy in the book?

❏ Yes, please credit this remedy to:

_____

❏   No, please use my remedy, but do not use my name in the book.

Either way, yes or no, if I use your remedy, I'll send you a free copy of the new edition of home remedies.

Your remedy can be one which uses cinnamon, or simply one that you feel others would like to know about.

My favorite chapter in *The Cinnamon Book* is:

_____

_____

The most helpful remedy I appreciated in *The Cinnamon Book* is:

_____

_____

_____

_____

_____

What I liked best about *The Cinnamon Book* is:

_____

_____

_____

_____

_____

_____

_____

_____

Would you be interested in hearing about my new cook-
book when it becomes available?

_____

My name and mailing address is:

_____

_____

_____

If you have any comments or experiences to add to the
information you've read in this collection, or if you have information for subsequent editions, please address your letters to:

Emily Thacker
PO Box 980
Hartville, OH 44632

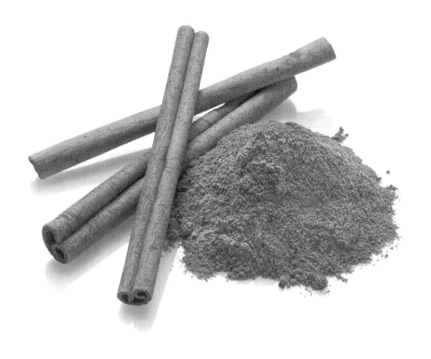

---- ✂ please cut here ----

The Cinnamon Book

90-DAY MONEY-BACK GUARANTEE

□ **YES!** Please rush _____ additional copies of The Cinnamon Book and my FREE copy of the bonus booklet "*Secrets of Pep, Vim and Vigor At Any Age*" for only $19.95 plus $3.98 postage & handling. I understand that I must be completely satisfied or I can return it within 90 days for a full and prompt refund of my purchase price. The FREE gift is mine to keep regardless. *Want to save even more?* Do a favor for a close relative or friend and order two books for only $30 postpaid.

I am enclosing $ _____ by: □ Check □ Money Order (Make checks payable to James Direct, Inc.)

Charge my credit card Signature _____

Card No. _____

Name _____

Address _____

City _____ State _____ Zip _____ Exp. date _____

Mail To: JAMES DIRECT, INC. • PO Box 980, Dept. CIN125 Hartville, Ohio 44632 • http://www.jamesdirect.com

Use this coupon to order the "The Cinnamon Book" for a friend or family member -- or copy the ordering information onto a plain piece of paper and mail to:

The Cinnamon Book
Dept. CIN125
PO Box 980
Hartville, Ohio 44632

Preferred Customer Reorder Form

Order this...	If you want a book on...	Cost...	Number of Copies...
Garlic: Nature's Natural Companion	Exciting scientific research on garlic's ability to promote good health. Find out for yourself why garlic has the reputation of being able to heal almost magically! Newest in Emily's series of natural heath books!	$9.95	
Amish Gardening Secrets	You too can learn the special gardening secrets the Amish use to produce huge tomato plants and bountiful harvests. Information packed 800-plus collection for you to tinker with and enjoy.	$9.95	
The Vinegar Book	Apple Cider Vinegar's magical mix of tart good taste and germ killing acid. Vinegar has more than 30 important nutrients, a dozen minerals, plus vitamins, amino acids, enzymes — even pectin for a healthy heart. And, there are hundreds of cooking hints.	$9.95	
The Vinegar Home Guide	Learn how to clean and freshen with natural, environmentally-safe vinegar in the house, garden and laundry. Plus, delicious home-style recipes!	$9.95	
Emily's Disaster Guide of Natural Remedies	Emily's new guide to infectious diseases & their threat on our health. What happens if we can't get to the pharmacy – or the shelves are empty, *what then?* What if the electricity goes out – *and stays out?* What if my neighborhood was quarantined? How would I feed my family? Handle first aid? 208 page book!	$9.95	

Any combination of the above $9.95 items qualifies for the following discounts...

| | | **Total NUMBER of $9.95 items** | |

Order any 2 items for: **$15.95**

Order any 3 items for: **$19.95**

Order any 4 items for: **$24.95**

Order any 5 items for: **$29.95**

Order any 6 items for: **$34.95** and receive 7th item

FREE Any additional items for: **$5 each**

FEATURED SELECTIONS

		Total COST of $9.95 items	
The Magic of Baking Soda	*Plain Old Baking Soda A Drugstore in A Box?* Doctors & researchers have discovered baking soda has amazing healing properties! Over 600 health & Household Hints. *Great Recipes Too!*	$12.95	
The Honey Book	Amazing Honey Remedies to relieve arthritis pain, kill germs, heal infection and much more!	$19.95	
The Magic of Hydrogen Peroxide	An Ounce of Hydrogen Peroxide is worth a Pound of Cure! Hundreds of health cures, household uses & home remedy uses for hydrogen peroxide contained in this breakthrough volume.	$19.95	
The Vinegar Anniversary Book	Completely updated with the latest research and brand new remedies and uses for apple cider vinegar. Handsome coffee table collector's edition you'll be proud to display. ***Big 208-page book!***	$19.95	

Order any 2 or more Featured Selections for only $10 each... | **Postage & Handling** | $3.98* |

| | **TOTAL** | |

* Shipping of 10 or more books = $6.96

90-DAY MONEY-BACK GUARANTEE Please rush me the items marked above. I understand that I must be completely satisfied or I can return any item within 90 days with proof of purchase for a full and prompt refund of my purchase price.

I am enclosing $_____ by: ❏ Check ❏ Money Order (Make checks payable to James Direct Inc)

Charge my credit card Signature _____

Card No. _____ Exp. Date _____

Name _____ Address _____

City _____ State _____ Zip _____

Telephone Number (_____) _____

❏ Yes! I'd like to know about freebies, specials and new products before they are nationally advertised. My email address is: _____

Mail To: **James Direct Inc.** • PO Box 980, Dept. A1219 • Hartville, Ohio 44632
Customer Service (330) 877-0800 • *http://www.jamesdirect.com*

©2013 JDI A209IM

GARLIC: NATURE'S NATURAL COMPANION

Explore the very latest studies and new remedies using garlic to help with cholesterol, blood pressure, asthma, arthritis, digestive disorders, bacteria, cold and flu symptoms, and MUCH MORE! Amazing cancer studies!

- -

AMISH GARDENING SECRETS

There's something for everyone in *Amish Gardening Secrets*. This BIG collection contains over 800 gardening hints, suggestions, time savers and tonics that have been passed down over the years in Amish communities and elsewhere.

- -

THE VINEGAR BOOK

Emily Thacker's collection of old-time remedies has hundreds of ways to use vinegar for health & healing, cooking & preserving, cleaning & polishing. See how vinegar's unique mix of more than 30 nutrients, nearly a dozen minerals, plus amino acids, enzymes, and pectin for a healthy heart has been used for thousands of years.

- -

THE VINEGAR HOME GUIDE

Emily Thacker presents her second volume of hundreds of all-new vinegar tips. Use versatile vinegar to add a low-sodium zap of flavor to your cooking, as well as getting your house "white-glove" clean for just pennies. Plus, safe and easy tips on shining and polishing brass, copper & pewter and removing stubborn stains & static cling in your laundry!

- -

EMILY'S DISASTER GUIDE OF NATURAL REMEDIES

Emily's most important book yet! If large groups of the population become sick at the same time, the medical services in this country will become stressed to capacity. *What then?* We will all need to know what to do! Over 307 natural cures, preventatives, cure-alls and ways to prepare to naturally treat & prevent infectious disease.

- -

THE MAGIC OF BAKING SODA

We all know baking soda works like magic around the house. It cleans, deodorizes & works wonders in the kitchen and in the garden. But did you know it's an effective remedy for allergies, bladder infection, heart disorders… *and MORE!*

- -

THE HONEY BOOK

Each page is packed with healing home remedies and ways to use honey to heal wounds, fight tooth decay, treat burns, fight fatigue, restore energy, ease coughs and even make cancer-fighting drugs more effective. Great recipes too!

- -

THE MAGIC OF HYDROGEN PEROXIDE

Hundreds of health cures & home remedy uses for hydrogen peroxide. You'll be amazed to see how a little hydrogen peroxide mixed with a pinch of this or that from your cupboard can do everything from relieving chronic pain to making age spots go away! Easy household cleaning formulas too!

- -

THE VINEGAR ANNIVERSARY BOOK

Handsome coffee table edition and brand new information on Mother Nature's Secret Weapon – apple cider vinegar!

* Each Book has its own FREE Bonus!

All these important books carry our NO-RISK GUARANTEE. Enjoy them for three full months. If you are not 100% satisfied simply return the book(s) along with proof of purchase, for a prompt, "no questions asked" refund!

10362303R00118

Made in the USA
San Bernardino, CA
13 April 2014